D1253585

Popular Medicine in Seventeenth-Century England

Popular Medicine in Seventeenth-Century England

Doreen Evenden Nagy

Bowling Green State University Popular Press
Bowling Green, Ohio 43403

Copyright © 1988 by Bowling Green State University Popular Press

Library of Congress Catalogue Card No.: 88-70523

ISBN: 0-87972-435-8 Clothbound
       0-87972-436-6 Paperback

Cover design by Gary Dumm and Greg Budgett

For John Mark, Steven, Peter and Nancy

Acknowledgements

This book had its inception in a graduate thesis supervised by Dr. J. D. Alsop to whom a great debt is owed, not only for suggesting the topic, but for his scholarly, consistent and kindly guidance. Thanks also to Patricia Yates-McShane and Michael McShane for their help and encouragement and to the staff of Mills Memorial Library, McMaster University for their invaluable assistance. Finally, I wish to acknowledge the financial assistance rendered by the Ontario Graduate Scholarship Program and McMaster University.

Doreen Evenden Nagy
Hamilton, Ontario

1988

Contents

Introduction

In a recent article "Some Current Trends in the Study of Renaissance Medicine," Nancy Siraisi has demonstrated the tenacity with which historians of European medicine continue to cling to the perspective of the medical "profession" when examining health care between the years 1300 to 1600.[1] Although Siraisi briefly acknowledges the work of Margaret Pelling, whose local studies on sixteenth-century East Anglia have demonstrated the remarkable diversity in training and background of medical practitioners, she urges historians to renewed investigation of the "Latin learned tradition."[2] Siraisi also points out various primary sources, all of which are related to physicians, which she feels should be explored in order to gain insight into the "scientific ideas" of the period.[3] Siraisi's views are typical of the "Whiggish" interpretation which medical historians have traditionally favoured but which has recently been called into question, not only by the work of Margaret Pelling, but by medical historian Roy Porter. Porter has challenged the concept of a "medical Enlightenment" in eighteenth-century England and concluded that more attention should be paid to the layman rather than the medical professionals or "scientific medicine" in any assessment of Englightenment medicine.[4]

A glance at the work done by most of the medical historians of seventeenth-century England supports many of Porter's eighteenth-century perspectives. Aside from Pelling's work (which extends to 1640), medical historians have ignored the role of non-professionals in the delivery of health care. R.S. Roberts has concentrated on licensed professionals both in London and the provinces; his particular interest was the way which surgeons and apothecaries moved into the general practice of medicine.[5] John Raach's pioneering study has attempted to locate physicians practising in the provinces in the first half of the century.[6] Charles Webster, whose impressive work *The Great Instauration* contained a lengthy section on seventeenth-century health care, while not always complimentary to the professionals, nonetheless devotes most of his discussion to the licensed practitioner.[7] Medical historian Walter Pagel concentrated on the 'great names' in seventeenth-century medicine, producing studies of Paracelsus, Harvey and Van Helmont.[8]

1

Other topics traditionally favoured by medical historians include the education and training of medical personnel as well as studies of the professionalization of medicine.[9] Robert Frank concluded that a small medical elite existed which became progressively enlightened as the century progressed.[10] Medical historians have in general popularized the view that the profession as a whole attained new levels of competence and knowledge, especially in the second half of the seventeenth century.[11]

Despite this single-minded concentration on the role of the professional, Pelling and Webster concluded a recent study of sixteenth-century medical practitioners with the observation that a system of health care existed which was "largely independent of the services of medical graduates".[12] The present investigation will focus on this system of health care which was sustained by non-professionals.

The first task of the researcher who undertakes a study of popular, alternative, complementary or fringe medicine is one of definition.[13] Who were the professionals? Where should the boundaries separating "popular" from "official" practitioners and practice be set? For some historians, such as Sir George Clark, the history of medicine is the history of the Royal College of Physicians, an approach which eliminates the problem of definition.[14] Christopher Hill neatly avoided identifying the "medical profession" in his lengthy discussion entitled "The Medical Profession and its Radical Critics."[15] Matthew Ramsey, on the other hand, clouded his discussion of popular medicine in nineteenth-century France with unwieldy terminology such as "illegal healers," "itinerant quacks," "sedentary healers," "illegal practitioners" and "unauthorized practitioners".[16] Pelling and Webster have included in their designation of "medical practitioner," any individual whose occupation is basically concerned with the care of the sick."[17] Their definition embraces a large number of practitioners traditionally excluded from studies and also discounts contemporary value judgements of a pejorative nature. In this respect, their view is supported by Roy Porter who pointed out the difficulty in distinguishing between "proper medicine" and quackery.[18] While there is much to recommend Pelling and Webster's approach to a definition which is cognizant of the realities of early modern English medical practice, this paper will focus more narrowly on the non-professional practitioner, and hence a more selective definition is warranted. Inasmuch as the present study argues for the absence of any clearly defined method of practice or corpus of knowledge which was peculiar to unlicensed practitioners, our definition will attempt to deal with popular practitioners, rather than popular medicine per se. Seventeenth-century medical practice in general was an untidy mixture of folklore, superstition, Galenic theory, herbal tradition, astrology and, eventually, chemical medicine. Into this mélange, both licensed and unlicensed practitioners indiscriminately dipped. To this end, then, all of those practitioners with a university education and/or episcopal license to practice physick, or those with an affiliation with an apothecary's or surgeon's guild will be considered professionals.[19] All others, including highly skilled but self-taught empirics, will be classed as popular practitioners.

My purpose in this thesis is to study the nature of popular medicine with a focus upon particular features of this larger theme. It will be argued that economic and geographic factors, among others, played a prominent role in ensuring the reliance of the majority of the English population upon the services of popular practitioners. The religious milieu of the period, moreover, encouraged and reinforced this reliance. It will be shown that popular practitioners used the same treatments as the professionals to treat a broad spectrum of ailments and achieved similar results. And, finally, as a case study of a large and vital segment of popular practitioners, it will be demonstrated that women of all social groups played a prominent and characteristic role in popular health care throughout seventeenth-century England. The result should be a better informed, albeit somewhat altered perception of seventeenth-century English health care.

Chapter I
Geography and Medical Practice

R.S. Roberts has argued that the principle of supply and demand worked against the unlicensed practitioner early in the seventeenth century and that "the popular but amateur clerics, their wives and other local wise people were increasingly displaced from practice."[1] In this instance, he cited as an example the increasing access of apothecaries to new and more exotic drugs against which the simple herbal treatments of local traditional healers failed to compete. Thus, Roberts' argument presupposed the availability of this more sophisticated alternative to major segments of the English population. In many areas of England, however, throughout the seventeenth century, sick and dying individuals were denied access to treatment by a member of one of the recognized "healing professions." One of the factors which contributed to this situation and which nurtured the existence of unorthodox or unlicensed practitioners was the geographic isolation of many areas and the difficulty of travel.

Medical historians such as Roberts have traditionally ignored the realities of geographic distribution, particularly in the provinces. But geography imposed severe limitations on the services which licensed practitioners could reasonably provide. In many areas the demand for medical services far outweighed the supply of licensed practitioners, despite Roberts' contention that unlicensed practitioners were increasingly displaced by practitioners with more qualifications. When Raach concluded, as a result of his pioneer study of medical practitioners in the provinces, that people had "well-trained doctors by their standards to provide for their needs," he failed to take into account the fact that there were over 9,000 parishes in England at the time.[2] If each of the 814 doctors in his study had practiced for the entire forty-year period which Raach examined, each one would have been responsible for the health needs of at least one hundred parishes in order to support Raach's contention that the population in the provinces had access to "well-trained" practitioners.[3] In the year 1600, London, with 30 Fellows of the Royal College of Physicians and 20 candidates and licentiates, boasted the largest number of physicians of any urban area; although approximately 100 surgeons and 100 apothecaries were located there,

4

only one physician was available for every 4,000 inhabitants.[4] By 1639, however, each Fellow or licentiate of the College would have been responsible for almost 10,000 inhabitants according to Christopher Hill. Robb-Smith has also estimated the number of medical graduates per population at one per 10,000 during the first half of the century and one per 6,000 during the latter half of the seventeenth century.[5] With sickness and death widespread throughout the century, unlicensed or popular practitioners were an absolute necessity in order to bridge the huge gap between the services provided by professional practitioners and the needs of the population.

Even though the actual supply of authorized practitioners in London was grossly inadequate for the population as a whole, there was the perception that superior care was available in London. One of the reasons that treatment in London was preferred was the fact that it eliminated many of the uncertainties (created by long distances and poor roads) which faced the physician. Lady Margaret Hoby and her husband Sir Thomas were willing to travel 150 miles from their home in N. Yorkshire to take "physic" in London early in the seventeenth century.[6] Surgeon Simon Harward who published a treatise in 1602, noted that in London "the people enjoy a great blessing of God in having so many worthie and expert Phisitians dwelling together."[7] Harward felt that this fact ensured good treatment around-the-clock unlike the situation in the country where the absence of qualified practitioners in many areas resulted in bad treatment by unqualified (if well-meaning) practitioners. In 1640, Sir William Playters, aware of the difficulties entailed in obtaining medical care in the country, petitioned the king for permission for his wife and himself to remain in London in order to continue treatment with their physician.[8] The Barrington family encouraged Judith Barrington to seek treatment in London in 1630 for an undisclosed ailment simply because she would be assured of daily visits by a skillful physician, for at least a week.[9]

Norwich, with the second largest urban population in England, claimed nineteen physicians in the years 1603-1643, which was the largest number for any provincial town.[10] Aside from these licensed physicians, recent study has revealed the necessity for, and extent of, popular medicine as it was practiced by a large number of unlicensed practitioners.[11] Not only did doctors tend to congregate in the larger centres of population such as London and Norwich, a disproportionately large number settled in areas like Bath in order to supervise the taking of "spaw" waters for a variety of ailments.[12] For example, Raach lists eleven licensed practitioners at a time when the population of Bath was only 2,000; this translates roughly into 190 inhabitants per practitioner, a rate which is astonishingly low when compared with that of London.[13]

In 1653, Robert Pierce, a physician who settled in Bath for personal health reasons, encountered problems because the town had too many physicians. He was forced to draw his patients from well outside of Bath and to travel "for Ten or Twenty, sometimes Thirty miles about".[14] As soon as some of the older doctors retired, Pierce was able to practice in Bath.

Not only did Bath experience an over-supply of physicians at the expense of other parts of the country, in some cases practitioners abandoned their practices in other counties to accompany and supervise patients at Bath, thus sacrificing the needs of the many to the demands of the few (usually of the upper class). Dr. John Hall described how Dr. Lapworth, a colleague who usually practiced at nearby Warwick, prescribed for Mrs. Wilson of Stratford-on-Avon while she was at Bath.[15] Tobias Venner undoubtedly hoped to derive monetary rewards from the seasonal flood of well-to-do clients to Bath each year. He noted that he was a "Doctor of Physick in Bath, in Spring and Fall, and at other times, in the Borough of North Petherton near to... Bridgewater in Somersetshire."[16] There is abundant evidence from seventeenth-century records that the great majority of men and women who made the pilgrimage to Bath were from the affluent segment of society.[17]

In addition to the problems created by a qualified medical force which was numerically inadequate and badly distributed, bad roads and inefficient methods of transportation made the delivery of medical services difficult, if not impossible in many cases, and encouraged the continuation of more traditional forms of medical treatment at the hands of local, unlicensed practitioners. Provincial roads, especially those which were frequently travelled, were scarred by deep ruts which became almost impassable in rainy weather when they became muddy quagmires. At dusk, the roads became virtually invisible, limiting travel time in the winter to a few hours. At the best of times, the physician-on-horseback could cover twenty miles a day.[18] As late as 1685, a diplomat travelling on the great route to Holyhead took five hours to cover fourteen miles: much of the time he walked while his lady travelled in a litter.[19]

Up until 1670, physicians with a thriving practice rode sidesaddle through the streets of London on elaborate "foot cloths" which hung to the ground, gaudy symbols of the prestige and high status of the rider.[20] By 1670, especially in London, it was becoming customary for physicians to make their visits in a carriage, but this additional expense resulted in a extraordinary increase in the fee which the physician charged.[21] Dr. William Denton, a London doctor who frequently travelled to the provinces to treat various members of the Verney family, attended his patients on horseback until 1652 when he decided to have a coach (he was then about 45 years old). Even so, he found travel difficult and experienced frequent delays when accidents occurred. For example, when

Denton travelled to Cheshire for a relative's confinement, several of his horses became lame; by the time Denton arrived, Betty Alport had been delivered.[22]

Coach travel proved more comfortable, but a coaching advertisement from 1673 which boasted of "one day" service between London and Oxford failed to note that more than sixteen hours of travel were required to cover the fifty-seven miles separating the two cities; the variable of bad weather increased the trip to two days between Christmas and Lady Day (March 25).[23]

Medical literature of the period contains references to the difficulty of obtaining professional medical treatment outside of major towns or cities. As early as 1550, Humfrey Lloyde in his forward to "The Gantle harted Reader" indicated that his translation of the early works of Hippocrates, Galen and Auclen was intended for use "in tyme of necessity when no lerned Phisicion is at hand."[24] The renowned Richard Banister, "Chyrurgion, Oculist and Practitioner in Physicke," published a treatise on diseases of the eyes in 1622.[25] In setting forth his qualifications, he noted his long experience and constant travel about the country to treat those suffering from eye diseases. He also listed his reasons for travelling about: he could see "more bad eyes in one month than in halfe a year at home"; the publicity he gained in outlying areas would give him fame at home, and finally, many poor people were unable to travel a distance to get the help they needed.[26] Banister wrote of his testimonials from various centres; two which he mentioned were signed by the magistrates of Lincoln and Bury St. Edmonds.[27]

In 1634 Richard Hawes wrote "My full intent and desire is to give direction to the poore and plaine people, such as cannot (for their remote living) get a chirurgion."[28] Hawes also gave instructions for preparing "an excellent salve, and easy to make, fitting for every Country man to have in his house."[29] Thomas Millwater's treatise *The Cure of Ruptures* was published in 1650. In it, Millwater claimed that he had to travel as much as one hundred miles to attend to patients. Given the condition of roads and the method of transportation, it is highly unlikely that many patients with ruptures were able to avail themselves of his services.[30] In *A Treatise Concerning the Plague and the Pox*, published in 1652, the author, one A.M., noted the value of the medicines contained within which were recommended for "a necessitous time and in places remote, both from able Phisitians and Chirurgions."[31] Also in 1652, Nicholas Culpeper published an English translation of Galen's *Art of Physick*. In his forward to the reader, he listed his reasons for attacking the monopoly of medical knowledge which the College of Physicians was attempting to enforce. One of his reasons, he gave as follows:

Hiding the Grounds of Physick murders all such poor wretches as die either through want of an able Physitian neer, or through want of Knowledg of such medicenes as grow neer them or for want of knowledge of the true method of Physick.[32]

Richard Elkes, "student" of physick, published a treatise in 1651 which he directed to soldiers as well as country people because he had seen "many men" lose their lives not only through carelessness and ignorance, but because there was no physician or surgeon at hand to treat them. Elkes included information for the preservation of health in addition to the usual assortment of cures, intended for lay use.[33] In 1656, Robert Turner translated a work by friar Moulton which he also enlarged and published. His declared purpose was to enable people to treat themselves in surgical emergencies, including broken bones. Turner particularly commended his work to country people, since he noted the dearth of surgeons (especially good ones) in the country.[34]The same year saw the publication of *A Compleat Practice of Physick* by John Smith. He noted that his work was intended for those who by reason of "distance of place cannot conveniently repair to a Physitian."[35] As late as 1689, physicians were writing of the "problems" encountered by "country people who, lying at a considerable distance from physicians" were compelled to use the services of non-professionals.[36]

Although not an accredited physician, the highly influential and widely-read Robert Boyle published a book in 1688 entitled *Medicinal Experiments: or a Collection of Choice and Safe Remedies. For the most part Simple and easily Prepared: very useful in Families, and fitted for the service of COUNTRIE PEOPLE.*[37]In the author's preface, Boyle added: "The most of these receipts are intended chiefly for use of those that live in the country, in places where physicians are scarce, if at all to be had, especially by poor people."[38]

In 1658, a treatise by Plenis de Campy was translated and published in England. This work is important because it is an illustration of how Hippocratic teachings still influenced the way in which physicians carried out their practice of medicine. De Campy offered advice on treating medical "crises." He advocated that the doctor remain with the patient throughout the time the "crisis" was developing, usually a period of five days. De Campy stressed that this phase could not be rushed and stated that this was the reason Hippocrates maintained that a physician should have "but a few patients."[39] Hippocrates' advice seems to have been taken seriously by many seventeenth-century physicians who spent long periods of time with a single patient. When travelling time was added to the long period which physicians remained with patients, other potential patients were left without the assistance of a qualified practitioner for weeks, even months, creating a powerful incentive to the development and maintenance of alternative forms of treatment.

In the light of De Campy's treatise, Dr. William Denton's attitude toward Lord and Lady Wenman was understandable. Although not treating a "crisis," by twentieth-century standards, he felt compelled to remain with them at Thame Park once they were launched on a course of physick in 1657, even though he had to neglect his busy London practice. He explained:

My Lady was purged yesterday and my Lord vomited to-day and untill I have settled them, I cannot with any conveniency stirre any whither.[40]

Some years earlier, Denton had refused "a great deale of money to goe but fivety miles out of towne" to treat a patient because he could not spare what he reckoned as ten days away from his practice.[41] Although on that occasion Denton served the interests of his London patients, both incidents illustrate the fact that London patients competed with patients in the provinces for the doctor's attention, the losers being forced to seek alternative solutions to medical problems.

The diaries and correspondence of private individuals living at various times throughout the seventeenth century provide numerous insights into the difficulties imposed by distance when health problems developed. Lady Margaret Hoby lived in the tiny village of Hackness, N. Yorkshire, early in the seventeenth century. As the closest centre where a physician could be found was York, some 35-40 miles distant, it is not difficult to understand why Lady Hoby took an active part in treating the ailments of people living in the surrounding area. Lady Hoby described the case of a child born at Silpho who had no anus and whose parents brought him to Lady Hoby. She wrote "I was earnestly intreated to cutt the place to see if any passage could be made, but although I cutt deepe and searched, there was none to be found." Not only was there no physician nearby, in this case "Lady Hoby was probably the only surgeon" in the area."[42] When Lady Hoby and her husband wanted "preventive" physick, they travelled to York or London. In October 1600, when they travelled the 150 miles to London, Lady Hoby was also seeking attention for a painful, abscessed tooth.[43] Although the Hobys were affluent enough to solve the problem of professional medical care by undertaking lengthy journeys, there were times when Lady Hoby was forced to find other solutions. On several occasions, she treated herself: "...and then I was busie about a dressing for myself...beinge before not well."[44] When Lady Hoby had an acute illness, which she described as "a fitt of the stone," she stayed in bed for a week while her mother came to stay with her.[45]

There were other well-to-do families living in the country who only partially solved the problem of access to qualified medical practitioners. Lady Joan Barrington of the prominent Essex puritan family employed the services of two physicians at various times in the years 1628-32. Thomas

Burnet was located at Braintree, 14 or 15 miles from the Barrington estate at Hatfield, Broad Oak in Essex. Perhaps this distance proved a problem in obtaining emergency treatment, or perhaps Dr. Burnet was frequently away meeting the needs of other patients. At any rate, Lady Joan also used the services of John Remington of Great Dunmow, which was only half the distance of Braintree from the Barrington estate, even though Remington is not known to have been a professionally qualified physician.[46]

In 1630, Jane Hook, Lady Barrington's niece, wrote to her aunt from her home in Clatford, Wiltshire, and described how she was obliged to travel fourteen miles to "Salesberry" and "lye at a friends house of his [her husband] and there take phisick."[47] The Salisbury practitioner however, did not start a trend and doctors continued to travel to their prosperous patients. In January 1637, Dr. Edmond Randolph of Canterbury rode ten miles to the Oxinden estate in Barnham, Kent, to treat a family member who was ill.[48]

Mr. Wakefield, a prosperous importer and friend of Sir Ralph Verney, described how a horsesmith in the town of Edmonton, Middlesex, had successfully treated members of his family and "many others." Wakefield vouched for the excellence of the smith's care and explained:

Physitians of quality. . .cannot spend any tyme with us; and the trouble of sending soe far too and again, besides of ten tymes the mistakes and miscarriages of things, forces us to doe that which if we were in London, we should hardly venture upon.[49]

Although Edmonton was less than ten miles from the City of London, Wakefield felt that it was better to use the services of a horsesmith than to face the problems created by distance which could result in rushed or bad treatment. When Mr. Butterfield, a clergyman from Sir Ralph's parish in Claydon, Buckinghamshire, tried to get medical advice for an ailing parishoner by having Sir Ralph contact Dr. Denton in London, the woman (Mrs. Taylor) became understandably impatient. She consulted an unlicensed practitioner at nearby "Bucks," much to the vicar's chagrin.[50] Dr. Robert Wittie had practices at the centres of York and Hull. In 1652, he left his patients and rode the fifty miles to Hipwell to treat Alice Thornton who was seven months pregnant and threatening to miscarry after a hazardous trip. He remained a week with her thereby depriving the patients at both his home areas of his services for almost two weeks.[51]

Ann Murray, the future Lady Halkett, became dangerously ill while staying at Naworth Castle, Cumberland, in 1649 as a guest of Sir Charles Howard and his wife. Her hosts sent to Newcastle in Northumberland, approximately forty miles away, to fetch a physician "butt he being sicke could not come, butt sentt things which proved ineffectual."[52] The dilemma which faced the Howards can only be fully appreciated when viewed in the context of Raach's study which revealed that the entire county of Cumberland could claim only one qualified physician in the period up to 1643; he was located at Newbiggin.[53]

The correspondence of Lady Brilliana Harley of Brompton, Hereford, to her son Edward, a student at Oxford, revealed the difficulty of getting medical attention from physicians who lived at a distance.[54] The Harley family used the services of Dr. Charles Deodati who resided at Chester in the years 1608-1638, a city which lay about thirty-five to forty miles from the Harley estate.[55] In April 1639, at least three days after the doctor was summoned to attend to her husband, she wrote "I thank God, your father is reasonabell well. Dr. Deodati is not yet come, nor the messenger returned. Antony Childe went for him on tuesday last."[56] Ten days later, she again wrote to her son, noting that when the doctor finally arrived and treated her husband, he had no time to attend to her personal medical problems. The following year, Lady Harley complained again that Dr. Deodati had just left Brompton after treating her husband, and had suggested that she also take "preventive" physick and blood letting. She had, however, refused his offer since she felt it was wrong to take treatment unless she was actually ill, even though it was virtually impossible to get treatment from Dr. Deodati when it was needed.[57] Lady Harley's undisclosed symptoms were probably not life-threatening, but her dilemma illustrates the fact that, in many cases, wealthy individuals living in the country could not obtain professional medical treatment when they wanted it.

In the same year, the Harley family began to call on the services of Dr. Nathaniel Wright, newly incorporated as a Doctor of Physick at Oxford, whose training encompassed study at Cambridge and Bourges, France. Dr. Wright lived at Shewsbury, Salop, about 27 miles from the Harleys.[58] In May 1640, Lady Harley wrote to her son that Dr. Wright had been there for a week to treat Edward Penner, a servant on the Harley estate. Later that year she told him that Wright "took much time" treating Mrs. Yats, a resident at Brompton.[59] In March, 1640, Mr. Ballam tried to contact Dr. Wright to come to Brompton and treat him but the doctor was away in Glocestershire.[60] It is noteworthy that Wright would have had to travel a minimum of 50-60 miles in order to treat a patient in Glocestershire. A month later, Brilliana Harley reported that Mr. Ballam was by now "very ill," but that the doctor would come "the following munday."[61] In April 1642, Doctor Wright came to the estate and stayed with Edward Harley's cousin for three or four days until he was well on the road to recovery from a serious illness.[62] On another occasion, Wright visited Robin Harley, Lady Harley's young son who was recovering from an illness: the doctor made this call on his way back from treating a patient in Worcestershire, approximately forty to fifty miles from his home in Shrewsbury, Salop.[63] Although the Harleys were able to make use of the doctor's services on frequent occasions, Dr. Nathaniel Wright was the only licensed physician in the entire county of Shropshire, a fact which indicates that the majority of the residents of the area would be forced to depend on the services of unlicensed practitioners.[64]

When Lady Ann Clifford's husband was en route to Buckhurst in 1617, he became so ill, he was compelled to stop several times and go into houses along the way where he received assistance from the occupants, no physicians' services being available.[65] In 1626, Sir Nathaniel Bacon had coughed up blood before leaving London. He then planned his trip home so that he could pass through a town (Colchester) where he knew that there was usually a physician, in case his condition worsened.[66] This illustrates the problem which faced travellers of the day when so few parishes could claim the services of a physician.

In 1653, General Blake was forced to come ashore when he became ill and disembarked at Walderswick near Southwald; the report sent to the Admiralty Committee described a situation familiar to many rural inhabitants:

This place affords no accommodation at all for one in his condition, there being no physician to be had here abouts, nor any to attend him with necessary applications.[67]

In her introduction to *The Household Account Book of Sarah Fell of Swarthmoor Hall*, Alice Clark emphasised the isolation of Swarthmoor; in order to get supplies, it was customary to dispatch a servant across the Sands at low tide for the difficult and sometimes dangerous fourteen mile trip to Lancaster.[68] Under the circumstances, it is easy to understand why family members, as late as the 1670s, became adept at treating themselves, their servants and their neighbours in this remote region of Cumberland. In the five years covered by Fell's meticulously-kept record book, there is no record of a payment to a medical practitioner. In December 1674, a payment of four pence was noted for the delivery of a letter from Richard Lower, noted London medical practitioner, to his brother Thomas Lower, husband of one of Sarah Fell's sisters. This letter probably contained advice for Thomas's wife who subsequently miscarried.[69] In addition to the isolation of Swarthmoor, Raach's study of country practitioners failed to locate any doctors in Lancaster up to 1643. In the entire county of Cumberland he found only one practitioner, while the neighbouring county of Lancashire had four or possibly five practitioners, all located at Manchester.[70]

The isolation of the Essex parish which Ralph Josselin served for more than forty years was probably a factor in the selectivity with which physicians' services were utilized by the Josselin family. Josselin's diary is filled with comments about frequent illness for which no doctor was in attendance. The Josselin family usually treated themselves or sought help from various parish residents. In 1645, when the midwife was needed, Josselin went to a neighbour who had offered to fetch her. The neighbour's horse was out of the pasture, causing some concern until it was found. This probably indicated that Josselin himself, at that time, did not own a horse.[71] By 1676, Josselin's fortunes had improved and he rode to his surgeon on several occasions when he needed treatment for a chronic leg ailment which he had unsuccessfully tried to treat with a variety of home remedies.[72] Toward the end of his life, Josselin, unable to obtain relief near at hand, sent to London for advice. Dr. Cox obliged by sending various prescriptions to Josselin. About the same time, in 1683, Mary Josselin went to London to be "lett blood," indicating that when professional services were needed, they were often unavailable in small rural communities, as late as the 1680s in the more advanced home counties of England.[73]

The relatively short distance of two and one half miles could prove disastrous when emergencies arose, given the methods of transportation and the condition of seventeenth-century roads. In January 1658, John Evelyn of Says Court, Deptford, Kent, described how his son Richard, aged five, experienced six "fitts of the Quartan Ague" with symptoms of "hot fitts and sweates." Evelyn sent to London for physicians while the child was still alive, although desperately ill:

but the river was frozen up and the coach broke on the way ere it got a mile from the house; so as all artificial help failing, and his natural strength exhausted, we lost the prettiest and dearest child.[74]

Dr. Wells and Dr. Needham, two London physicians, arrived after he was dead and carried out a post-mortem the following day.

Sending for a doctor who resided at a distance was uncertain, especially when doctors were frequently away for long periods of time treating other patients. This fact must have encouraged both the use of lay practitioners and of home treatment. For example, Alice Thornton called Dr. Wittie to treat her daughter Joyce in January 1666 when she was ill with fever and red spots on her face; later in the year, when daughters Katherine and Naly had smallpox, they were treated by "brother Portington." When son Robert had the same deadly disease, he was attended by Hanna Abelson and Margery Millband with no mention of a physician.[75] Her customary physician was probably unavailable when Lady Anne Clifford's beloved eldest daughter was so ill in 1617 that her mother feared her life. Although Lady Clifford recorded the doctor's attendance a month later, for this first of a series of severe "fits of the ague," the mother was forced to cope with her daughter's symptoms.[76]

An examination of available doctors' records from the period is valuable for giving additional insights into the way geography affected medical practice. One of the earliest descriptions of a doctor's practice originated within the boundaries of the North-Riding of Yorkshire. The name of its author is unknown, but the area covered by his practice is fairly well defined by the records which he kept for the years 1609 and 1610.[77] Most of his patients came from an area roughly bounded on the north and south by Thirsk and North-Allerton (approximately 8 miles), and on the east and west by Rydale and the Swale River (approximately 15 miles). In many cases, the doctor rode 15 miles to attend a patient; on occasion he rode the additional 10 miles required to see a patient at Richmond.

The importance of travel in the practice of medicine was illustrated by the petition of John Wyndebank, M.D. to Parliament in 1650. He requested that the restriction which ordered him to practice within a five-mile limit be lifted. It was virtually impossible for a physician to confine his practice to such narrow limits and his request was subsequently granted.[78]

Many of the limitations of professional provincial medical practice in early seventeenth-century England can be illustrated by reference to Dr. John Hall who carried on an active medical practice in Stratford-on-Avon spanning the years 1600-1635. Several outlying areas which also claimed his services on occasion were: Whitlady Aston, at a distance of 20 miles from Stratford; Aven Dasset, 14 miles; Knowle, 15 miles; Warwick, 9 miles; Pillerton, 8 miles; and Quinton 7 miles.[79] It is difficult to ascertain from the selected case studies in Hall's book (some 178 were chosen by Hall for publication out of a possible one thousand or more cases), how often Hall visited the 25 or so outlying areas which he mentioned. He was a very busy doctor who, for instance, visited the Earl and Countess of Northampton, some 40 miles distant, twice in one month. He mentioned at least two instances when "much business" prevented his personal attendance on patients.[80] It would be fair to say that, in most cases, visits to outlying areas were undertaken to treat patients who were acutely ill, like Mrs. Sheldon of Grafton and Lady Rouse of Rousenlench who both suffered complications of child birth, or patients who had chronic illnesses which other "cures" had failed to relieve.[81] In the latter categories were Mrs. Delaberr of Southam who could not retain her food and Doctor Thornberry, Bishop of Worcester, described as "long tormented with a Scorbutic Wandering Gout," who had been wrongly diagnosed by another physician.[82]

When Hall attended Mrs. Hanberry at Worcester, he travelled 25 miles each way, while treatment for Joan Chidkin of Southam required a round trip of 34 miles on horseback.[83] When Hall visited Lindlow Castle, four or five days were spent in travelling in addition to the time necessarily spent administering treatment. Hall's records of his patients' illnesses include a description of his own medical problem, a severe case of bleeding haemorrhoids which were aggravated by horseback riding.

Despite this, Hall wrote: "Yet daily was I constrained to go several places to Patients."[84] When Hall finally became disabled for a lengthy period, no mention was made of another physician to carry on his practice. Moreover, existing records fail to show any other qualified physician in Stratford-on-Avon at the time; the closest known practicing physician was Francis Phipps at Kenilworth, some 14 miles away.[85]

In at least one instance, Hall acknowledged that he was unable to fulfill his obligations personally. Mrs. Jackson, about twenty-four years of age, succumbed to post partum fever and "a grevious Delerium." Hall noted that "By reason of much business I could not have time to visit her, yet their was happy success by the following Prescriptions." He then outlined various purges, applications and bleedings, the latter to be carried out by the local surgeon. He concluded "and thus in seven days she was happily cured."[86] On another occasion, Hall's treatment of an acutely ill woman, also suffering from a complication of childbirth, was interrupted, and the patient almost died: "Multitude of business calling me away, and hindering my return to her, she sent again to me, telling me she had like to have been suffocated with Phlegm the night before."[87] In addition to his professional duties, Hall was elected to the town council in 1632 and the demands of town business clashed with those of his patients. On at least one occasion, Hall was fined for non-attendance at a council meeting which he missed in order to treat Sid Davenport of Bushwood.[88]

The Bedfordshire Historical Record Society published another remarkable collection of the case records and correspondence of a seventeenth-century physician in 1951.[89] John Symcotts' practice (which he began about 1620 and carried on until 1662), covered a wide area in Huntingdonshire and Bedfordshire and extended into Northants, Cambridgeshire and Hertsfordshire. A number of patients lived as far as 25 miles away from Huntingdon, the town where Symcotts practised for forty years, until his death in 1662.[90] In 1649, Symcotts travelled to Faldo to treat Mistress Jane Crouch, a trip of almost 28 miles. Unable to lodge at her house, he stayed at Mr. Tavener's house, a mile from where his patient lived, until she had been successfully treated.[91] At various times he travelled 20 miles to treat Mr. Cater of Kempson, 25 miles to Ampthill to treat the Franklin child,20 miles to Hinskworth where Mr. Hanchet lived, and 15 miles to Thurleigh where his patient Col. Herby lived.[92] Because of the heavy demands of his practice, Symcotts employed the services of an assistant, Gervase Fullwood, whose medical qualifications are unknown.

One of Symcotts' patients of longstanding was Richard Powers, a coal merchant living at Ramsay, about ten miles from Huntingdon. Symcotts was unable or unwilling to make the trip to Ramsay in response to Powers' frequent requests for advice on medical matters. Instead there was a lively exchange of letters between doctor and patient, Powers being billed for the prescriptions and instructions which Symcotts sent.[93] Powers could also consult a local practitioner, possibly a barber-surgeon, whom Symcotts describes as "a wandering practitioner, your doctor there" and whom Symcotts accused of giving bad advice.[94] The lines of communication between Powers and Symcotts were frequently interrupted by Symcotts' absences and Powers was forced to accept advice from Fullwood, Symcotts' assistant. In 1636 Symcotts was absent when Powers requested his help; Fullwood responded "the doctor is from home." As to the treatment which he suggested, Fullwood added the proviso "If this will not do, send for the doctor again."[95] In June 1639, Fullwood was obliged to respond to Power's request for help and he wrote, "I am sorry to hear you are so ill. The doctor is not yet come home." Fullwood stated that he had taken upon himself to send something "though but a little--and that very easy" until he could consult with Dr. Symcotts about Powers.[96] Some time later, a different problem in communication arose with Dr. Symcotts sending an apology to Powers. He explained that "The letter which you sent me on Saturday was not given me (though at home) till Monday at noon."[97]

Symcotts' correspondence with his patients vividly depicted the problems which faced families confronted with the twin spectres of illness and death, but none more poignantly than the undated letter of Rebecca Holgate. She wrote:

Worthy Sir,
My son has bled again since you were with us and I much fear the night. Therefore I humbly desire your advice what we had best do as to opening again, or whatever else you please. Your humble servant...[98]

Although it is obvious that this mother believed that her son would be dead before morning, she was aware that he had already had as much attention as she could reasonably expect from a busy practitioner with a widely scattered practice. The only professional assistance she could hope for now was a word of advice transmitted by a third party.

The Rutland manuscripts contain portions of the personal accounts of Lord Roos (Ros) of Belvoir Castle, Lincolnshire. In them we find that Mr. Alston, "physicion," was paid £6 in December, 1607, for attending Lady Roos at Belvoir, about 19 miles from his home base in Nottingham. Between November 1614 and August 1616, Dr. Rydgeley of Newark travelled on four occasions to Belvoir Castle approximately 44 miles away. In one instance, he spent six days at the castle for which he was paid £6. In December 1614, he spent ten days at Belvoir treating the Earl of Rutland, or Lord Roos, for a fee of £10. Taking into account the doctor's travelling time, this last occasion deprived his other patients of his services for at least two weeks, a fact of some significance inasmuch as Rydgeley was the only known physician practising at Newark at that time.[99]

Unlike the peripatetic Hall and Symcotts, the astrological physician Richard Napier treated thousands of patients from his home in Great Linford, Buckinghamshire, in the years 1597-1634.[100] Although in Napier's case, the patient and not the physician made the trip, the variable of distance remained a significant factor in determining the number of people who resorted to his services. MacDonald shows that the number of patients which Napier treated from any given area "was inversely proportional to the distance they had to travel to reach his home."[101] Napier had acquired the reputation of someone who could effectively treat individuals displaying symptoms which today we would associate with mental illness. As highly sought after as his skills may have been, the problems related to seventeenth-century travel circumscribed the boundaries of his direct contact with patients.

Alexander Read, who lived in the period 1580-1641, trained as both a physician and surgeon. After obtaining his M.A. in Great Britain, he travelled to the continent to study surgery under the great Ambrose Pare. He was incorporated at Oxford and created a Doctor of Physic in 1620. One of the most eminent practitioners, writers and medical lecturers of his time, Read did not confine himself to one locale. Instead, for many years he moved about the Midlands and western part of England as well as along the Welsh border. From cases which he cited in his writings, it is clear that he practiced in Denbigh and Chester and as far afield as Tavistock and Bath.[102] Read may have been motivated by a desire to serve as wide an area as possible or perhaps to gain experience in treating unusual cases. Bath was well-supplied with doctors at this period and Chester could boast of at least one outstanding physician; Read possibly offered some form of consultant service.[103] Whatever his motives, permanent residents of the area which he visited would, in the long term, reap few benefits from this type of practice and would be ultimately dependent on other avenues of medical treatment. That Read was well aware of the problem faced by people living at a distance from towns or settled areas is indicated by his endorsement of a work by Owen Wood published in 1651 for the use of laymen "where neither Physicians nor Apothecaries can be had."[104]

Somewhat later in the century, the diary of John Causabon casts light on the activities of a busy surgeon described as "a general practitioner with special skill in accidents and injuries."[105] The diary covers periods in the years 1668-1669 and 1674-1690 and gives details of Causabon's practice in Canterbury, Kent, and the surrounding area. The treatment of surgical cases and accident victims was often more time-consuming than the treatment carried out by physicians using standard medical procedures. When Causabon accidentally cut an artery instead of a vein in an attempt to "bleed" a patient, he was obliged to pass a week at the patient's house and for three days and nights was on twenty-four hour duty in order to save the patient's life.[106] At another time an eleven-year-old boy from Cornwall, some 260 miles from Canterbury, came to Causabon's home where he boarded while undergoing treatment for a chronic ulcer on his thigh.[107] In 1678 Causabon travelled more than six miles to Chilham to give "emergency" treatment to a child bitten by a "viper or adder."[108] At Chilham, also, Causabon treated Goodwife Gilbert for "Dropsie" and "Scurvie."[109] In 1681 he ministered to the wife of Colonel Rooke, governor of Dover Castle at St. Lawrence, some fourteen miles away. In 1682, he was sent for again by the Colonel whose "cure" involved numerous "difficulties and inconveniences" for Causabon.[110] By 1683 the doctor was experiencing severe financial difficulties and could no longer afford a horse. Because travel was indispensable to the active practitioner, Causabon resorted to borrowing a succession of horses which he described as" "cook's mare," "Downing's little black mare," "Sears bay mare," "Mother Tadd's mare."[111] On one occasion John Gilbert of Chilham sent a man and two horses so that the doctor could visit Gilbert's bed-ridden wife.[112]

Most of the evidence regarding seventeenth-century medical practice comes from the segment of society with the means to pay for the services of licensed practitioners. It is important to understand that even this group was only partially successful in overcoming the obstacles of distance and time in obtaining professional assistance.

When we return to the diary of a mercer's apprentice who lived in Ashton in Makerfields, Lancashire, and covered the years 1663-74, we are afforded a rare glimpse into the lives of ordinary people living in the provinces.[113] Roger Lowe, who could read, write and reckon, was an exception in an age when few men of his station possessed literacy skills.[114] His services were in great demand in an area extending eight to twelve miles in all directions from Ashton. Roger wrote letters, drew up wills, indentured apprentices and carried out a myriad of clerical tasks. Roger's diary reported many events which occurred in the small communities which he visited, including the important events of life and death. He was called to read scripture at the bedside of the dying and was a faithful mourner at many funerals. Although Roger's diary is full of reports of death (as well as illness), there is not a single mention of a formal medical practitioner. Perhaps James Corles of Winnick who pulled the tooth of Roger's friend was one of the unofficial practitioners in the small town where he lived.[115] Roger expressed great interest in a rhyme which reportedly staunched blood if repeated three times; he recorded it in his diary as a self-help measure in case of injury.[116] However, it seems certain that even as Roger's skills were utilized in the role of "unofficial notary," there were men and women whose healing skills were called upon in the frequent medical emergencies which were a part of daily life in seventeenth-century England.

Although scholars such as D.C. Coleman have recently argued that men and women living outside of urban centres have tended to experience mental as well as physical isolation, a fact which would reinforce the rejection of "outside" medical intervention in favour of local resources, Roger's diary does not support this view.[117] Roger himself travelled on numerous occasions to Manchester and Chester. Perhaps more tellingly, when the inhabitants of Ashton were canvassed to help the victims of the Great Fire in London in 1666, more than half of them contributed.[118] A more likely explanation for the absence of licensed practitioners in Roger's diary was the fact that there were either no practitioners close enough to consult, or, if they did exist, they lay well beyond the economic resources of this segment of society. Raach's directory showed that two practitioners had practised at Manchester, (approximately twenty miles from Ashton) earlier in the century, while two other physicians had resided even further away.[119] This was a total of four practitioners for the entire county of Lancashire. Although Roger visited Chester in neighbouring Cheshire county to attend fairs and listen to organ music, the sole practitioner at that centre, Dr. Charles Deodati, left in 1638 and was probably not replaced.[120] In the final analysis, the fact that only 415 provincial parishes out of over 9,000 could claim the services of a resident, fully qualified practitioner, argues strongly for the fact that the bulk of the population, whether affluent or poor, depended on non-professionals in the treatment of illness.[121]

Chapter II
The Economics of Seventeenth-Century English Health Care

It has been estimated that up to half the population of seventeenth-century England lived in or near poverty at various times, while another 30-35% were able to maintain themselves only slightly above the poverty line. The links between poverty and ill-health have been well-established: for approximately 85% of the population faced with chronic ill-health as well as frequent acute illnesses, the traditional or popular method of treating disease was the only viable alternative.[1]

Although a small percentage of the "settled poor" lived in towns which provided some sort of medical treatment for those who qualified for poor relief, relatively few town corporations offered these services. Those that did, such as Norwich, Newcastle, Chester, Ipswich and Barnstaple, hired practitioners with a wide diversity of background and training. The most detailed study to date involves Norwich in the late sixteenth century. Here it has been shown that the group from which the town hired its "official practitioner, who was responsible for treating those on poor relief, was made up of women surgeons and healers (approximately one-third of the group), barber surgeons, surgeons, bone-setters, apothecaries, physician-surgeons and other tradesmen who also practiced physick."[2] Of the seventy-three practitioners in Norwich in the years 1570-1590, only five, or less than 7%, were university-trained. This fact demonstrated that academically qualified practitioners formed only a tiny minority in the overall picture of medical care, including the provision of care to those on poor relief, a trend which extended well into the first half of the seventeenth century. Medical services were frequently provided by the keepers of lazar houses and poor houses. These services would again fall into the range of treatment known as popular or traditional, since the keepers of these houses were not usually licensed practitioners. Occasionally, a lazar keeper did have some training; one such, Lawrence Wright, was a barber-surgeon who treated approximately twelve patients in Norwich from June 1615 to June 1616, a figure which represented a tiny fraction of the sick poor residing in the city at that time.[3]

Hospital services were completely inadequate for treating the masses of sick poor. London, with a population of 500,000, could boast of only four hospitals, the largest two of which, St. Bartholomew's and St. Thomas', provided only three hundred beds between them. Charles Webster has pointed out the strains which the Civil War placed on the hospitals which tried to cope with large numbers of wounded soldiers. Webster notes that St. Bartholomew's and St. Thomas' as well as Christ's Hospital and Bridewell failed to meet their prewar levels of treatment until the 1650s, creating a situation which pitted increasing demand against decreasing availability of services.[4]

In Norwich, the largest of the provincial towns, the main hospital (St. Giles), became a negligible factor after 1620 when seriously ill patients were sent home and infectious cases were refused.[5] As with many of the main provincial centres, it was not until the 1770s that "adequate" hospital care was provided with the establishment of the Norfolk and Norwich General Hospital.[6]

The standard study of early modern English philanthropy has shown that outside of London, only a very small percentage of charitable donations went for the support of hospitals and other care of the indigent sick.[7] In the county of Norfolk, for example, the total was merely 0.42% of all charitable bequests. The policy of issuing a license to individual paupers to collect money to pay for unusually costly treatments or cures had generally fallen into disrepute by the end of the sixteenth century; some licenses were still being used in the late seventeenth century to finance expensive treatment in at least one major provincial town. This form of "licensed begging," was, however, unsystematic and completely dependent on "individual application and individual generosity."[8]

Evidence of what professionals charged "ordinary" people for treatment is limited. In addition, in assessing the capacity of the vast majority of men and women to meet the demands of payment to licensed medical practitioners, it must be borne in mind that during the first three decades of the seventeenth century, the average wage rate of a skilled building craftsman was twelve pence a day, while for a labourer in the same trade it was eight pence.[9] By mid-century, their respective rates had increased by approximately one-third. Despite this increase, A.L. Bier argues that the working poor got poorer between 1500 and 1650 as the increase in living costs "outstripped wage rates by a factor of two to one."[10]

In the first half of the seventeenth century, London physicians charged 6s 8d to 10s for a visit, a fee well beyond the means of all but a small group of prosperous patients. Moreover, Christopher Hill has pointed out that the high fees which London practitioners charged their patients were the result of a deliberate attempt by the College of Physicians to restrict the number of Fellows and licentiates of the College to ensure that fees could be kept high.[11] Dr. John Symcotts, a practitioner in the provinces, probably charged 2s 6d for consultations; in addition, his patients paid substantial apothecaries' bills such as those recorded for Mr. Powers, a prosperous coal merchant who frequently used Symcotts' services.[12] Early in the century, a surgeon in the North-Riding of Yorkshire usually charged a shilling for a vomit or purge and 2s 6d for more complex treatments. On occasion, he accepted payment in food or drink; one woman gave him fish worth 8d in exchange for advice while one of his prosperous patients gave him "3s worth of 'wine and good perry' for letting her blood."[13]

Another surgeon practising in the provinces, John Causabon, charged 2s 6p in the last half of the century "for a night call to a distance" over and above any charge for medicines. On occasion Causabon took into consideration the poverty of his patients; in one case he did not prescribe "Diette Drinks," in order "to save charges," even though he felt they were necessary to his patient's cure.[14] In this case inferior medical treatment resulted from the patient's financial disability.

In his study of the astrological physician Richard Napier, MacDonald found that Napier's standard fee of 12d, which included medicine, enabled all but an "indigent minority" to avail themselves of his services.[15] Nobility were charged more because they usually lodged at Napier's residence accompanied by one or two servants. According to MacDonald, Napier's popularity rested, in no small measure, on the fact that he charged such low fees at a time when the rich were the customary users of physician's services.[16] Although 12d was a very reasonable fee, it did constitute the daily wage of a skilled labourer. What must also be considered is the fact that many of the sick had already experienced prolonged unemployment due to ill health. In addition, the expense of travelling to Napier, plus loss of wages for those able to work, or those accompanying a sick relative, increased the cost of treatment. For these reasons, MacDonald's assumption that only an "indigent minority" were deprived of Napier's services can be questioned.

Examples of sums paid by Londoners of unknown occupation for medications used to treat illness include: £1.6.6 for three month's treatment of veneral disease in 1642; eleven shillings for a ten-day treatment of female hysteria in 1643; 15s 6d for liniment, clysters, etc., on three occasions between May 6-9, 1642; £1.6.10 expended over six occasions for the treatment of a case of diarrhoea, also in 1642.[17] Later in the century, sums paid by "ordinary" people to apothecaries included six shillings for two bottles of elixir and one shilling for six pills paid by a soap boiler's wife in 1673. Benjamin Fleetwood, a mason, paid thirteen shillings for two bottles of medicine and eight pills needed for one treatment in the same year.[18] In 1672, Mr. Russell, a baker, paid 16s

6d in August and a further 13s 6d in October for medication while Mr. Parris, a cloth dyer, paid £1.8.0 in apothecaries charges.[19]

Although doctors themselves left few records of what they charged, seventeenth-century manuscripts and documents provide some indication of what the well-to-do members of society paid for treatment at the hands of physicians, surgeons and apothecaries. Book-keeper's accounts, spanning the years 1604-1670, attest to the fees which successive Dukes of Northumberland paid for medical care. In 1604, £20 was paid for Lady Roos' treatment, and in 1605, £30 for the same Lady's treatment at Bath under Dr. Sherwood's supervision. For a three-month period in 1614, Lord Roos expended more than £32 in doctor's and apothecary's fees. In 1652, Lord Roos paid £20 to Dr. Prudian and £9.50 to Dr. Turnor. Two accounts from the 1660s show payments of £5 to a surgeon, Dr. Harris, and £4.5.0 to "Dr." Bacon, an apothecary. Early in the seventeenth century, the treatment of the Duke of Northumberland's "strained foot," a relatively minor ailment, netted a royal surgeon £4 and a Scottish surgeon £2. Sir John Gell paid a surgeon £13.9.0 in 1646 for "curing his neck wound."[20]

Sir Robert Cecil, Earl of Salisbury, paid £62.2.8 to an apothecary for the thirteen-month period between Aug. 1604 and Sept. 1605—an indication that reliance on professional medical treatment could cost £60 yearly in medicines alone.[21] When Paul D'Ewes, esquire, one of the six clerks of chancery, was treated by two London physicians, he was charged 20 shillings per visit and both Dr. Gifford and Dr. Baskerville visited twice a day.[22]

William Denton, himself a physician, paid more than £100 for costs incurred in the treatment of his two stepchildren, one of whom died.[23] The same doctor noted that Sir Ralph Verney paid him £30 in 1647 for delivering Sir Ralph's wife.[24] Sir George Wheler became ill shortly after dining at Dr. Denton's house on Christmas Day, 1655, resulting in medical expenses of £100.[25] Denton also reported on the incomes of other doctors: Dr. Radcliffe's "regular" fees netted him at least £4,000 per annum, while Dr. Mead's annual income was estimated at £5,000—£6,000. The most eminent physician of the mid-seventeenth century, Dr. Theodore Mayerne, left an estate of £140,000, according to Denton.[26] Later in the century, the fees rose even higher as the guinea (21 shillings) made its appearance in 1663 and doctors quickly appropriated it as the unit on which they based their fees. In 1687, Edmond Verney, son of Sir Ralph Verney, paid a surgeon three guineas daily for two weeks treatment to his injured arm.[27]

Grateful patients of wealth and means on occasion granted a doctor a lifetime annuity such as the one described by a Dr. Wiseman in 1660:

This person retired into the country [after his cure] and returned to London at the end of two years and acknowledged to me his cure by settling thirty pounds a year upon me during his life and paid me sixty pounds for the two years passed.[28]

Medical historians Poynter and Bishop have pointed out, moreover, that it was "not unusual in the case of rich and noble patients," to pay medical fees of 250 and 500 guineas and that records reveal that on one occasion, a practitioner prescriber a "purge" which must have been spectacularly successful; he was paid £65 for it .[29] It is clear, therefore, that regular professional medical treatment was beyond the means of the great majority of the English population, and that it was to the financial advantage of trained practitioners to direct their services toward those most ready and willing to pay lucrative fees.

An examination of seventeenth-century medical literature reveals a variety of responses by the doctors themselves to the question of medical treatment for those without money to pay for their services. Some merely acknowledged the existence of the problem; others suggested that doctors should treat the poor out of charity, while a third group published medical treatises, ostensibly designed to help lay people understand the nature and treatment of common diseases in order to treat themselves if they could not afford the services of a recognized or licensed practitioner. Before accepting the latter as proof of the doctor's good-will, the low literacy rate of the majority of the population must be taken into account.[30] David Cressy has demonstrated the link between social rank and literacy in his study of Tudor and Stuart England. For example, Norwich in the years 1580-1700, claimed a fully literate clergy and professional class while only 2% of the gentry were illiterate. On the other hand, the poor labouring class was 85% illiterate. It can be seen, therefore, that those most in need of medical advice of a self-help nature were those with the highest rates of illiteracy.[31] Moreover, there is reason to believe that at least some of the authors published their medical tracts for motives more concerned with profit than charity.[32]

William Clowes, one of Queen Elizabeth's surgeons, published a treatise early in the seventeenth centry on the cure of *Struma*, the open wounds which resulted when a tubercular abscess opened and became a chronically discharging sore. Clowes felt that these could be successfully treated by surgeons and his book was intended for them. For the poor, Clowes described an alternative course, that of treatment by the "royal touch":

...a mighty number of her maiesties most Loyall subjects, and also many strangers borne, are daily cured and healed, which otherwise would most miserably have perished. For many of them (their poverty was such) were not able to pay but a very little or nothing at all for their cure.[33]

Clowes accepted the fact that if you were poor and could not pay for a cure, or could not avail yourself of the "royal touch," your fate was sealed: to perish "miserably." There is no suggestion that the young surgeon, to whom Clowes specifically addressed his tract, should consider a non-paying client deserving of his healing skills.

The Poore-Man's Plaster Box (1634), written by Richard Hawes, was addressed to the needy segment of the population. On the title page Hawes wrote: "published for the common good of (as) such as stand in need." Hawes acknowledged that the problem of obtaining treatment might stem from unavailability, but added "or else (dwelling where they [physicians] may be had) want means to pay them for their paines..."[34] Hawes described remedies which were specifically adapted to the needs and means of a poor man. For example, if a patient was so poor, he had "no bed to sweat in," a reasonable substitute would be to cover the patient up to the chin with horse dung (his head being covered with hay). Hawes noted that this method of causing a sweat was effective and cheap; he admitted that it was not "cleanly."[35] He also gave directions for a drink made of "dried earthworms," a low-cost treatment for a "poore man" who had sustained bruising, as well as other inexpensive and efficacious cures.[36] Hawes concluded his book with the observation that it was intended "for the poore and plaine man, not for the rich and learned,...an instruction for poore householders." Hawes, then, was writing not for the vagrants, almsmen and social outcasts of his era, but for the reasonably respectable, albeit poor, householders who he assumed would not have the means of availing themselves of professional medical services. It is also interesting to note that Hawes linked wealth and learning.[37]

Alexander Read's *Most Excellent and Approved Medicines,* which was published in 1651, claimed to offer advice for almost any medical or surgical contingency which might arise. Noting that in some cases, whole estates were spent on medicines, he pointed out that his book could "be had at a very cheap and easie rate: So that even the meane and poorer sort of people who for want of ability cannot go to the Physicians in time of Sickness and visitation" might get some help and advice from the small volume described as "precious jewel."[38]

Nicholas Culpeper was the most influential and widely published seventeenth-century critic of the monopoly exercised by the medical profession. A self-professed student of physick and astrology, he called forth the condemnation of the College of Physicians in 1649 when he translated the pharmacopaeia used by physicians and apothecaries from Latin into English. His professed purpose in translating the work was to enable the lay public to avail themselves of commonly used medicines and simples without the expense of consulting a physician. He condemned the avaricious practitioner:

Send for them to a poor man's house who is not able to give them their Fee, then they will not come and the poor creature for whom Christ died must forfet his life for want of money.[39]

The physician's responsibility toward the poor remained a primary, lifelong concern of Culpeper who discussed at length the qualities which he felt were essential to a good physician; the ability to display compassion toward the poor and treat them whether they could pay or not was one of the most important attributes a doctor should possess.[40] A few years after his early death, Culpeper's widow published his final work. In the forward was Culpeper's eloquent plea on behalf of the poor. He described how in many cases the medicine and cure for a common illness could cost one quarter of the patient's net worth. In other cases, a family was obliged to spend as much as would provide the basic necessities of life for a year.[41] Culpeper accused the medical profession of class discrimination:

Is Physick only made for rich men, and not as well for the poorer sort? doth it only wait upon Prince's Palace, and never stoop to the cottage of the poor? doth it only receive gifts of the King, and never thanks and prayers from him that hath only thanks and prayers to bestow?[42]

In the case of Sir Richard Carew, Oxford graduate and London practitioner, it is difficult to separate the elements of a physician's concern and an entrepreneur's zeal. Carew published a tract in 1652 extolling the virtues of "warming stones."[43] In it, Carew described the benefits of owning a "warming stone": since a poor man without a fire of his own could warm a stone at a neighbour's fire, it saved the cost of a fire, as well the dangers associated with a fire. Carew claimed that warming stones were effective for treating "colds of aged and sick, women in child bed and nursing and young children," as well as "cold fits of agues" and ruptures, colic, fluxes, toothache, blindness and deafness. His brief treatise closed with a list of patients who, Carew claimed, had benefited from using his stones. Finally, he gave specific directions as to where the stones (with their cases) could be purchased.

Thomas Brugis, doctor in Physick, emphasized the responsibility of the physician to treat poor patients, going so far as to say that "no disease is infectious to him," who treated these unfortunates. He predicted punishment from God would be meted out to doctors who were derelict in their duty toward the sick poor.[44]

In 1651, W. Bremer, who described himself as a practitioner in Physick and Surgery, published a book which Dr. William Turner had written in the mid-sixteenth century. Bremer described his motive for publishing it: "for the benefit of the poorer sort of people."[45] Seven years later,

John Tanner "student in Physick and Astrology," noted that his book, containing not only diagnostic techniques, but also descriptions of cures and medications, would be of particular benefit to those who lacked the financial resources "to confer with a Physitian." As a physician, Tanner believed that his book would save the lives of many who would otherwise die, since they lacked the resources of money and knowledge.[46] In *The Poor Man's Physician and Chyrurgion*, published in 1656, Lancelot Coelson, self-professed student in Physick and Astrology, offered directions for a variety of treatments including bleeding and tooth-drawing. His *Epistle Dedicatory* urged fellow practitioners: "let our Physicians not mind gain and self interest more than to be harboured under the roof of the poorest vassal in the world."[47]

Thomas Willis, one of the foremost physicians of his generation, extolled the use of the laurel leaf in 1666.[48] He urged its use as a medicinal agent which was safe, efficacious and available at no cost. Also included in the pamphlet were antidotes for the plague with several specifically directed to "the poorer sort." These were made up of readily available materials such as herbs, roots and weeds. A posset-drink made of butter roots boiled in "Pestilential Vinegar" was also intended for "the poorer sort;" for those with more money, Willis included an equivalent posset-drink made of more costly ingredients such as mithridate, salt or wormwood and syrup of citron.[49]

Another dimension to the issue of the high cost of medical treatment was introduced by the rise of the Paracelsians or chemical physicians in the 1650s and 1660s. These practitioners were proponents of a new form of medical theory and treatment which was far less complex than therapy based on traditional Galenic theory. Charles Webster has noted that because of its relative simplicity, the cost to the patient was lower and self-treatment was facilitated.[50] George Starkey was one of the most active proponents of chemical or Helmontian medicine. He commended his method to the reader as more simple and "less chargeable" and attacked his more traditional colleagues, who, he argued, continued to employ outdated and ineffectual methods of treatment for which they charged huge fees.[51] After discussing the high cost of medical education and a medical practitioner's license, Starkey argued that doctors, in turn, wanted to restrict the monopoly of medical practice to members of their own socio-economic group. Moreover, once a member of that profession, they would defend to the utmost a position "that cost them so dear." Finally, Starkey believed that most doctors were more concerned with fees than with the performance of their duties. He claimed that experienced doctors gave only one word of advice to fledgling physicians: "*Accipi Donum*, or Take your Fees".[52] Starkey described how the cure for a simple ailment was often prolonged into a "Fortnight's cure" in order to increase the doctor's fee. In some cases, the apothecary's bill was £5-£10 with an equal amount demanded by the physician "for what in the first place was a plain Diary."[53]

Starkey also indicted the apothecaries whom he accused of making a thousand percent profit on their wares.[54] He charged that the doctors connived with the apothecaries in order to bilk their wealthier patients; the doctor sent lengthy prescriptions (which included many expensive ingredients) to the apothecary, who "by secret agreement" substituted cheaper ingredients. The doctor was compensated by an annual fee for his part in the arrangement.[55] The archetypical "successful" doctor who earned £1500 annually and refused to treat poor people drew further reproach from Starkey.[56] The "fifteen hundred pound doctor" roused Starkey's ire, not only for his neglect of the poor, but also for cases such as that of a 'gentleman and his Lady' who paid £300 in apothecary's bills in connection with a short period of treatment by one such doctor.[57]

While Starkey's arguments were typical of the small group of men, inside and out of the College of Physicians, who supported chemical medicine, Nathaniel Hodges, M.D., was a staunch supporter of the medical profession's status quo (and the traditional Galenical school of medicine) who attacked illegal practitioners, especially empiricks,[58] He attempted to defend his colleagues against accusations of charging more than empiricks, for exactly the same type of treatment, by shifting the blame to the apothecary.[59] Hodges maintained that although in some cases the physician did not charge for his services, the apothecary overcharged the patient when filling the doctor's prescription. When exorbitant charges were made by the apothecary (as they frequently were), Hodges felt that the patient wrongly inferred some sort of collusion between the doctor and apothecary. Hodges, however, denied any complicity on the doctors' part and somewhat defensively asserted that all true physicians treated the poor without charge.[60]

Kitchin-physick or, Advice to the Poor by Way of Dialogue, was written by Thomas Cocke and published in 1676.[61] In it, the author stressed the importance of diet in the prevention and cure of disease. He noted in the 'Dedicatory' that the preservation of health and the prolongation of life were of particular concern to the "Poor of this Town, City and Country." Although Cocke criticized the unqualified practitioners whom he accused of administering treatments which frequently endangered the patient's life, he believed that people were driven to use the services of "quacks" or unlicensed practitioners because university-trained physicians withheld their services from the poor who could not afford to "pay both for advice and physick." Like Starkey and Hodges, Cocke suggested that the apothecary played a role in setting fees which were out of reach of the poor, and went as far as suggesting that the apothecary give the indigent patient money for food and medicine. Cocke himself claimed he used discretion in prescribing for a poor patient:

"I direct him (if any) no more Physick than is absolutely necessary; next I bid him keep a proper diet, or take a proper cordial against his diseases."[62]

Although Cocke was critical of both chemical and traditional physicians, he appears to have been influenced by some of the Helmontians' indictments against over-medication and avaricious apothecaries. For the sick poor, however, it made no difference whether the physician, the surgeon or the apothecary was responsible for the high cost of treatment - the end result was the same; the seventeenth-century sick poor were compelled to seek alternative forms of treatment which lay outside the domain of the establishment medical professions.

The perception that apothecaries were guilty of overcharging patients persisted throughout the remainder of the century and in 1703, Dr. R. Pitt, a fellow and censor of the College of Physicians published *The Craft and Frauds of Physic Exposed. The Very Low Prices of the Best Medicines Discovered...*(London, 1650).[63] In it, he listed approximately one hundred prescriptions and their prices with the comment that they were "herbs being mostly of English growth...commonly sold for one penny or less the handful." Pitt had earlier stated that both rich and poor "are pillaged of all their substance in every sickness by the excessive rates of their physic."[64] Although a professional himself, Pitt obviously felt that every man or woman should have access to home treatments at low cost, no matter what their income.

While some doctors were advocating consideration and charity, at least in print, there were others of entrepreneurial bent, such as male-midwife Peter Chamberlen, who claimed that when consideration was paid to the relative value of "Lives and Estates," as well as the cost of other operations, the true value of an obstetrical delivery to a well-to-do person was £100.[65] If the client had an estate of £1,000, he would accept a fee of £10. This fee could be further reduced upon presentation of a certificate by a minister or neighbour attesting to the fact that the patient's estate was less than £1,000.[66] Chamberlen's assertion that he accommodated patients of modest wealth was substantiated by Rev. John Ward, vicar of Stratford-on-Avon, whose diary covered a short period around the middle of the seventeenth century. Ward commented of Chamberlen: "his fee is five pounds, yett, I heard, if he come to poor people, he will take less."[67] At this time, however, the bulk of the midwifery practice was in the hands of women practitioners who customarily accepted modest fees for their services; this fact rather than professional charity may have accounted for Chamberlen's flexibility regarding fees. Even so, a fee of £5 would suggest that the patient's net worth was at least £500; if Chamberlen reduced his fee down to £1, the great majority of the population would still be unable to afford his services. This was a service intended for the elite; even a reduced fee was well beyond the reach of the average person.

While some doctors may have treated for a reduced fee, the records yield few examples of doctors who charged no fee to poor patients. John Causabon treated "a very poore man" for a draining abscess on his thigh for several years, apparently at no cost.[68] Thomas O'Dowd, author of the *Poor Man's Physician* was one of the few doctors who remained in London to treat plague patients until he himself succumbed to the disease in 1665. O'Dowd customarily treated poor patients who could not afford to pay for his services. His daughter, Mary Trye, took over his practice after his death and continued the tradition of treating the indigent.[69] Nicholas Culpeper, fiery critic of the medical profession, attended to forty patients daily, many of whom could not afford to pay, accepting only "their prayers" in return for treatment.[70]

An important and perceptive assessment of the position of the poor came from outside the medical profession when John Cooke, lawyer, published *Unum Necessarium or The Poor Man's Case*, in 1647. He outlined 12 recommendations for the benefit of the poor; the eleventh proposition urged "That Physicians, Chyrurgeons and Apothecaries might be assigned *in forma paperis*, as well as Lawyers, Attorneys, etc."[71] Cooke commented on high grain prices and low wages, noting that some poor men with a wife and three or four children were earning 6 pence daily; he pointed out the impossibility of such families living on 3 shillings a week. In some cases, physick could cost the price of more than a day's food.[72] Cooke felt that more doctors were needed and pleaded for an increase in their number, a view which directly opposed the monopolistic stance of the College of Physicians. He pleaded:

pray deal kindly with poore people when they are sick, for a poor man to give 10s for a visit, is as grievous many times as the disease itself: and yet life is sweet, Physick must be had at any rate; But some may better afford to give £100 for a cure, than others to give £5.[73]

Cooke noted that current medical thinking demanded that a doctor visit a patient three times a day and he noted with a fine touch of irony "how many people in this kingdom dye yearly, that can never get any Physitian to visit them in their sickness". Cooke added his voice to criticism of the apothecaries: "and how many pore people are there about London that had rather die then see an Apothecaries Bill."[74]

Cooke cited the example of Trigg the London shoemaker who had, it was claimed, successfully treated at least 30,000 patients over a ten-year period. Trigg was evidently a highly skilled and successful healer who compounded all of his medicine from "the best ingredients" and took "little or nothing from the poore, and from the rich 2s or 2s6." Trigg spent thirty shillings or more a week on Physick for the poor, but Cooke believed that apothecaries would sell the same ingredients at 500 per cent profit.[75]

Although Cooke condemned the apothecaries for their part in depriving the poor of access to treatment, he laid the blame on the doctors' shoulders by asking them for answers to four "queries": what do poor people do when the doctors flee to their country estates during epidemics; why do doctors not have supplies of drugs on hand to give to poor people; why do they write their prescriptions in Latin so people do not know what they are paying for; why do doctors not teach poor people how to concoct their medicines of herbs so that they can keep themselves in good health without the services of apothecaries and physicians?[76] As for Trigg's persecution by the College of Physicians who attempted to curb his practice by the levying of huge fines, Cooke suggested that the physicians were willing to sacrifice the well-being of poor people, who could afford no other form of treatment, on the altar of professional jealousy. The physicians were annoyed because Trigg had cured patients whom they had failed to cure.

Although the medical profession was quick to condemn the unlicensed and untrained practitioner on the grounds of ignorance and lack of skill, the profession tolerated, even approved of, the efforts of gentlewomen who treated the poor out of charity.[77] Early in the century, Richard Banister, renowned eye surgeon, condemned untutored women but approved of those like Lady Mildmay who treated the poor or

good mistris Dorrington of Godstow who would ever refuse to meddle with the rich, lest Art [the art of surgery] go unmaintained."[78]

Banister made clear that the medical profession had staked its claim to the paying patients, leaving to women of independent means the task of treating the sick poor "For love of goodness, not for hope of gain."[79] The medical profession then was intended, for the most part, to provide medical services for the wealthier classes who could sustain the substantial expenses of medical treatment. Popular practitioners drew the ire of the profession chiefly when they impinged upon health care for the elite.

Good evidence of the fact that licensed practitioners drew their clientele in the main from the small group who comprised five to fifteen percent of the population is found in the case records of Dr. John Symcotts and Dr. John Hall. In Symcotts' records, out of a total of 92 reported cases, 21 cases (23%) can be clearly identified with titled clients while another 64 (69%) were drawn from a group comprised of minor clergy (five cases), persons clearly associated with reasonably substantial land holdings (23 cases), merchants (2), skilled craftsmen, professionals and yeomen (7). Thus 85 cases which made up 92% of Symcotts' recorded practice were drawn from that segment of society which exercised some social standing and independence of livelihood.[80] Of the remaining cases, six (7%) came from a group with lower than yeoman status and only one client was described as poor (1.08%).[81]

Of the 177 cases in John Hall's records, 38 (21%) involved titled clients while another 122 (69%) were patients identified with an estate or other form of land holding (98 patients), the professions and skilled crafts (24 patients). The latter ranged from a bishop to a humble barber and included a female cooper as well as an apothecary's wife. It can be seen, therefore, that 160 patients or 90% of Hall's practice were drawn from the small group which could claim some sort of independent means and social position in local society. Only 16 patients (9%) lacked any designation and can perhaps be considered of status lower than yeoman. One patient "Hudson, a poor man" was so described.[82]

Table A

	Titled	Gentle-men and clergy	Undesig-nated	Poor
Symcotts	23%	69%	7%	1%
Hall	21%	69%	9%	0.56%

Note: Figures are approximate having been rounded off of the closest percentage point in most cases.

Symcotts' and Hall's practices show a surprising degree of similarity with regard to the socio-economic backgrounds of their patients (see Table A). Both doctors drew the bulk of their practice from titled clients or those with independent means associated with land holding, the professions or skilled crafts.

Undoubtedly the burden of ill-health weighed most heavily on the vast majority of the population who struggled to obtain the basic necessities of life. Medical fees were, however, also a grave concern for many members of society whose earnings placed them marginally higher than those at or below the poverty line. These included members of the minor clergy, some professions and those in skilled occupations. Mr. Belham, a tutor who resided on or near the Harley estate in Brompton, Essex, was typical of many who had a small amount of income to spare after their daily needs were met. Brilliana Harley wrote about Belham's predicament in March, 1640 after he had been very sick, possibly suffering from an "ague":[83]

but he is resolved to send to-morrow for doctor Rivit, but he fears he will stay longer with him than £3 will hould out, that he is willing to give, but can spare no more as he says; this 2 days he has been debating of, as they tell me; but now in this fitte, he resolves to send for him, and does not recken the charges.[84]

Captain Lovelace was able to afford treatment by Dr. Elliot for two weeks, after which time he was turned over to another doctor for treatment. A fellow practitioner perceived that the reason Dr. Elliot "tyred" of treating Lovelace was that he could no longer afford to pay for his treatment.[85] When John Causabon treated Mrs. Sprackling for widespread ulcers, he accepted £3, which he felt was only half of what he deserved for the two to three month "cure," but was all that the patient could pay.[86]

Ralph Josselin was the university-educated vicar of Earls' Colne, Essex, in the years 1641-1683. In the 1640s his family experienced many illnesses for which a physician's services were not sought. In 1645, his young daughter Mary was very ill "streyning and spitting up much blood." Josselin and his wife treated the child: "Mary continued ill, wee used meanes, the Lord Bless them."[87] Josselin's parish was experiencing hard times and in 1647 when he tried to collect the tithes on which his livelihood depended, there was nothing for the church: "people are bare," he wrote; "monye is dead."[88] On another occasion Josselin and his family had to live at Lady Honeywood's estate for eleven weeks because of personal poverty and on another occasion he admitted: "I was now without money."[89] Because of his financial problems, Josselin utilized the services of a medical professional, Dr. Francis Glisson, on only one occasion. Glisson, who was one of the most distinguished physicians of the century, was living less than ten miles from Earls' Colne at the time. He advised Josselin in 1649 regarding treatment of his chronically discharging navel.[90] When two of Josselin's beloved children were critically ill and died the following year, there was no mention of treatment by a professional. Eventually, Josselin's circumstances improved, he acquired some land of his own and the frequency of illness in the family decreased.[91] In later years, Josselin and his wife used the services of physicians, even to the extent of consulting a London physician, Dr. Cox.[92] Not only did the Josselin family appear to increase its use of professional practitioners as more money became available, Josselin was critical of Davy the butcher's wife who Josselin felt could afford medical treatment; instead, she paid a "poor" woman 2s to go to a doctor and ask for advice only rather than have him come or send a prescription.[93]

Although licensed practitioners drew the bulk of their patients from the group which included those having substantial landed wealth as well as members of the minor gentry, parish clergy, merchants, professionals and a small number of skilled craftsmen, members of this group had cause for concern in the expense of medical treatment. In December 1629, Sir Francis Harris, nephew of Lady Joan Barrington, wrote to his aunt requesting financial assistance because he had been forced to pawn his doublet and black hose in order to pay debts incurred by his "late dangerous sicknes."[94] James Oxinden of the wealthy Barham, Kent, family was obliged to write home in 1640 for a loan after a three-week illness had depleted his resources.[95] Several of the doctors themselves decried the fact that "whole estates" were spent on paying for medical treatment.[96] Dr. Denton, physician, noted that expenses incurred by family illnesses forced him "to sell my plate" to meet his debts.[97] Rev. John Ward reported another occasion when Doctor Wright, a London physician, accepted "sixty plates of silver" which were worth at least £150, in payment of his fee.[98] In 1660 Betty Verney, the sister of Sir Ralph Verney, was deeply in debt, partially because of expenses incurred through illness. Sir Ralph reported: "Physick keeps her very bare."[99] Another member of the Verney family complained: "if I sell myself to my skin, I must go along with my Husband to Oxford and have the opinion of a surgeon and a doctor both."[100] Further proof that the well-to-do found the doctor's fees burdensome, if not actually unreasonable, comes from Peter Chamberlen who criticized men of wealth who were unwilling to pay what Chamberlen claimed was a small percentage of their income for their wives' deliveries.[101] Walter Yonge, M.P. for Devon, found two London doctors "very high" in their charges to his neighbour, who worked in London.[102] John Causabon, surgeon, occasionally treated affluent patients such as Col. Rooke's wife, but he generally charged too little for fear of offending them and losing future "business," a fact which illustrates the attitudes of many of the wealthy clients toward their doctors.[103] Even the small group for which money should not have been a problem often perceived doctors' fees to be inordinately high, if not actually leading to hardship. For the vast majority of the English population, however, economic necessity dictated the only viable option when illness struck; self-help and treatment by traditional or popular practitioners remained the reality for seventeenth-century men and women in need of medical services.

Chapter III
The Intellectual Climate:
Religion and Popular Medicine

Sickness and premature death were commonplace throughout the seventeenth century. Indeed, many diaries and letters from the period are little more than chronicles of accident, ill-health and death.[1] Nevertheless, there is little evidence to suggest that the population as a whole rejected the services of traditional healers in favour of those provided by better educated or "scientific" professionals. One reason for this was rooted in the pervasive influence of religion throughout the period and, in particular, in certain aspects of religious belief. One indication of seventeenth-century preoccupation with religion can be found in a study by Judith Simmons which analyzed the publications of the year 1623; of a total of 327 publications, 120 were of a religious nature, 84 were on current events, often oriented to a scriptural interpretation, and 60 were educational books, which, for the most part, stressed piety and were "morally instructive."[2] Of 327 publications, therefore, 264 (80%) could be said to be explicitly or implicitly religious in nature.

Theologians stressed the necessity of accepting pain, illness and death as part of God's plan for man. The contemporary view that sickness and death originated with the Fall in the Garden of Eden, with the result that all subsequent illness became a visitation from God upon the transgressor, forged even more powerful links between spiritual and physical health. God was a divine judge who meted out punishment as he saw fit; therefore, it was to the realm of the spiritual one turned for healing.[3] The following examples will reveal the connections between spiritual and physical health in seventeenth-century England, and demonstrate why a relationship of this nature encouraged the retention of traditional medicine at the expense of professional medicine.

Edward Burghall, the puritan Vicar of Acton, expressed the views of his contemporaries in his diary which covered periods between 1628 and 1663.[4] Burghall saw life as a series of disasters which occurred as a result of individual, human sin. His is a dark and gloomy view of a punitive God who reacts to such simple pleasures as dancing on May

Day by striking a maidservant dead.[5] While Burghall has filled page after page of his diary with examples of God's wrath, he has given only one or two glimpses of a beneficent deity. Like others of his time, the vicar believed that the plague was a visitation upon a sinful populace. He noted that although the plague had killed many in various parts of the kingdom, "Cheshire was graciously preserved, where were many public fasts kept for the turning away of God's hand."[6]

In 1625, Robert Wright published *A Receyt to stay the Plague*.[7] This was not a medical tract; it was a sermon, like many others of this era, in which he urged "there is no such Physick as Prayer and Penitence, thereby to make an attonement between God and our sinnes."[7] He went on to say that God's mercy and grace were more powerful and efficacious than all of the herbs, drugs, simples and compounds in the world "for those soares that sinne doth make" and concluded that only by turning to God would the plague be lifted. Ralph Josselin, vicar of Earls' Colne, Essex, believed that the reason the toll from the plague was so high in 1665 was because "medicaments were used but no publique call to repentance."[8]

Nor was this view of the origins of the plague limited to the clergy. Thomas Mayerne was possibly the most renowned physician of his age; in response to the plague crisis of 1630, Mayerne advised that since God was "the first cause of all things, including the plague," the only sure way of escaping His "wrath," was "by prayer and a good life."[9] William Boraston of Salop, "Practitioner in Physick and Chyrurgery" published a treatise on the plague in 1641. In it, he described the plague as a punishment from God. Even so, he offered a number of "receipts" for the treatment of the plague which included the usual herbal ingredients, traditionally used against a whole range of ailments.[10] Significantly, he concluded his treatise by offering "a medicine for the Plague or for Sickness of the Soul" which began "Take a quart of Repentance" and went on to include all of the "ingredients of a godly life."

In 1655, Robert Bayfield, a physician who practised in Norwich, published a treatise which concluded that there could be no "general method of cure" for the plague since it was a punishment meted out in godly "rage." He did, however, list an assortment of readily obtained ingredients for those who wished to attempt a cure.[11] The same year (1655) saw the publication of a collection of medical and surgical addresses to Samuel Hartlib. At the end of one of the surgical treatises, there was a discourse on "Universal Medicine," which, the author argued, was to be found only in the "Kingdom of Christ."[12] As late as 1676, medical treatises, such as that by Thomas Cooke, which stressed preventive medicine, were appearing which advocated and above all things, devoutly invocate God for his benediction without which neither Paul, nor Apollo, Galenist nor Chymist, Food nor Physick can do anything[13]

In his diary, vicar Ralph Josselin chronicled on a daily basis the close relationship which he saw between ill health and personal short-comings. Josselin's prayers followed a pattern: thanks to God for his own and his family's health followed by a request for pardon of his sins in order to ensure continued good health. If there was illness in the family, Josselin saw this sickness, no matter how trivial, as a punishment for some transgression; this could be a sin of omission or commission. In 1644, when he and his wife suffered from heavy colds, Josselin believed that God was "exercising" them because "we have sinned this week."[14] When Josselin suffered with quotidian ague, he found greater relief from prayer than at the physician's hands.[15] At the delivery of her eighth child, Josselin's wife found that "the midwife did not do her part, but God did all."[16] In many respects, for Josselin's wife, surrounded by praying women, childbirth was more of a spiritual than a physical experience.[17] When Josselin's son was very ill in 1664, the family rejoiced because Dr. Collier, a friend, was staying with them.[18] Even so, Josselin did not fail to give God the credit for John's recovery.

The widespread interpretation of spiritual causes of ill-health found expression in the practice of faith healing in Stuart England. This could range all the way from unselfish humanitarianism, to quacks who exploited the prevailing climate of faith by using scripture. For example, on the one extreme was Valentine Greatrakes, the Irish healer who came to England at the behest of the prominent Conway family in an attempt to rid Lady Conway of her debilitating headaches.[20] Greatrakes refused to charge for his services, claiming that his power came from God.

On the other extreme was a practitioner such as Lewis Millwater whose qualifications are unknown. In 1650, he published *The Cure of Ruptures in Man's Bodie,* which was virtually an advertisement for a type of faith-healing.[21] Millwater stated that all illness was the result of sin but claimed that secondary causes produced ailments such as ruptures, which could be corrected. Millwater gave no details of how his "cures" were carried out, stating only that they involved no "cutting or lancing." Millwater gave his address and made the point that his cures could not be described in print, but must be personally experienced. Because of his choice of scriptures, which described miraculous cures by Christ and the apostles, Millwater probably used some form of laying on of hands accompanied by prayerful invocation of supernatural powers.[22] There is no question that Millwater's techniques involving positive thinking (or faith) could have resulted in the successful treatment of certain non-somatic ailments; however it is doubtful that his claims for legitimate cures of ruptures, which were his specialty, were substantiated.

Given the religious climate of early modern England, it was easy for the ubiquitous parish clergy, with their conviction that a sound soul ensured a healthy body, to slip into the role of healer. Indeed, in acknowledging the role played by the clergy as "common purveyors of medical lore," Charles Webster has cited the advice of Anglican churchman George Herbert who urged his colleagues to subsume the mantle of healer.[23] Throughout the century divines frequently performed in a dual capacity; some had medical degrees, others were self-taught. Phyllis Allen has looked at the group of men who obtained unearned medical degrees from the Church of England along with their studies in theology.[24] She has concluded that although this custom eliminated the prescribed courses in medicine, the recipients were possibly no worse as practitioners than their "logic-steeped contemporaries" who graduated from regular medical programmes.[25] Allen's conclusion shows how fine a line separated those practitioners who had the benefit of university medical studies from those who were (despite their university degree) virtually popular practitioners. Hugh Atwell, the parson of St. Ewe, was an outstanding example of the latter. A skillful popular practitioner and divine, he had gained a reputation as a healer noted for "the gentleness of his physick for his cures." Atwell based his regime on the administration of large quantities of milk rather than the harsh mixtures advocated by the Galenical school.[26] Richard Carew believed that Atwell had gained his knowledge from observing infants who were breast fed, an example of natural, as opposed to "formal," knowledge. Ralph Josselin attempted to diagnose a parishioner's illness on at least one occasion by viewing her urine.[27] Several years later, however, he was moved to express his relief that he had not gone beyond the limits of his calling; he had heard of the death of Mr. Whitings, the minister at Lexden, who had been bitten on the finger by a man with tonsillitis whom he had attempted to examine.[28]

Some divines, such as John Burgess (1563-1635) who obtained his M.D. and graduated from Leyden as well as Cambridge, were obviously highly qualified medical practitioners. Burgess carried on a medical practice as well as his duties as rector and preacher.[29] Edward Rogers was a divine who took specialized medical training when he was in his thirties to qualify him to practice medicine.[30] Rev. John Ward decided on a clergyman's career after completion of his university studies, but maintained a life-long interest in medicine, dabbling in it along with his clerical duties. Ward gave the names of five clergymen-practitioners in his diary which was full of snippets of medical information, but had very little by way of theological or spiritual content.[31]

At the other end of the spectrum was Richard Baxter, a well-known Puritan divine whose own bad experience with the medical profession as a young man encouraged his life-long interest in medicine.[32] Self-taught, he noted how his medical knowledge complemented his spiritual duties:

God made use of my practice of physick among them as a very great advantage to my ministry; for they that cared not for their Souls did love their Lives and care for their Bodies[33]

Even those divines who refrained from the actual practice of medicine frequently borrowed from the medical idiom to demonstrate the interdependence of medicine and theology. When Mr. Woods, the curate of Ashton, gave mercer's apprentice Roger Lowe "a healing receit for a diseased liver," there is no doubt the good clergyman believed it would have a physical effect. The lengthy receit began:

First fast and pray, and then take a quart of repentance of Ninivah and [pu]t nine handfuls of faith in the blood of Christ with as much hope and charitee as you can gett, and put it into a vessel of a clean conscience....[34]

The question for many was, however, what were the proper limitations or jurisdictions of medicine and religion? As early as 1612, the practice of combining professions in the church and in medicine drew criticism from members of the medical profession. John Cotta, a fully qualified practitioner who practiced in Northampton in the first half of the century, attacked "beneficed practicers" in his treatise on "Ignorant Practisers of Physiche," published in 1612.[35] Since many of the clergymen whom Cotta chastized were men of intelligence and learning, Cotta adopted the argument of "one calling" which he claimed was taken from the Christian view propounded by St. Paul.[36] Cotta repeatedly used religious arguments to support his charges:

...it is manifest, that this fluctuation of these men between two callings is offensive to God, scandalous unto religion and good men, and injurious unto commonweales, and but presumption borrowing the face of Divinitie.[37]

Despite the lofty tone of his charges, Cotta had no objection to divines who gave medical assistance to the sick poor (at no charge); he was concerned with those who charged for their services, thereby depriving "the more worthy of his fee."[38] Cotta tried to justify his claims on the ground that by attempting to carry out two professions, neither one was adequately sustained. The result, according to Cotta, was poor, even dangerous, treatment.[39]

In 1651 Dr. Robert Wittie (Doctor in Physick) translated and printed a work by physician James Primrose which contained criticisms of ministers or priests who practiced medicine.[40] Objections to the dual role were limited to a few members of the medical profession like Wittie and Cotta and had little or no practical effect.[41] Throughout England the clergy carried out traditional medical treatment as a service to their parishioners.[42]

Keith Thomas has argued that post-reformation religion not only brought about the decline of magical remedies for problems, it encouraged the use of self-help and prayer.[43] In the case of illness, Thomas' conclusion is well supported; the formidable combination of prayer and traditional remedies was widely adopted by non-professionals. Lady Warwick exemplified the devout gentlewoman who ministered to ailing relatives, friends and acquaintances.[44] She took special care, however, to provide spiritual remedies as well as the customary preparations from her 'closet' or 'still.' Lady Warwick placed spiritual health before physical well-being as did many of her contemporaries. It was this attitude which encouraged reliance on home treatment and spiritual exercises rather than recourse to professional healers. When she went to be with Lady Manchester in 1666, Lady Warwick stayed " 'till evening constantly watching all opportunities of doing her soul good."[45] When her sister was critically ill, the Lady's efforts were directed to helping her sister accept her illness a part of God's plan, an attitude which greatly weakened any inclination toward aggressive medical treatment by a professional.[46] On three or four occasions when her services were sought for desperately ill people (two of whom were probably stroke victims) Lady Mary used home medicines and prayer as well as sending a minister to visit the sufferer; no mention is made of a medical professional.[47] Lady Mary's husband suffered from painful chronic gout; her incessant efforts to convert him were intended as much to relieve his affliction as to restore his soul. Lady Warwick's priorities were clearly demonstrated by her description of her son's death from smallpox in 1664 when she closeted herself with him and did all she could for "his soul and body."[48]

Standing as he did outside of both the professions of the church and medicine, Robert Boyle, the esteemed philosopher and scientist, was probably representative of many educated men and women of his time with his views on sin and sickness, including the relative importance of the cleric and the physician:

...he who effectually teaches men to subdue their lusts and passions, does as much as the physician contribute to the preservation of their bodies, by exempting them from those vices...which are not enemies to man's life and health barely upon a physical account, but upon a moral one, as they provoke God to punish them with temporal as well as spiritual judgement; such as plagues, wars, famines...besides those personal afflictions of bodily sickness and disquiets of conscience, that do both shorten men's lives and imbitter them.[49]

Boyle concluded that the benefits derived from theology far outweighed those offered by medicine because the former dealt with aspects of life which endured forever:

...the benefits accruing from religion, may well be concluded preferable to their competitors since they not only reach to the mind of man, but reach beyond the end of time itself.[50]

Medical literature gives some indication of the fact that doctors were, in some instances, hard-pressed to justify their very existence in the face of prevailing seventeenth-century religious dogma. Early in the century, William Clowes acknowledged that the Royal Touch was a "divine" cure for scrofula. But beyond this, he contended that it was possible for the surgeon to use God-given gifts, which Clowes named "artificiall gifts," for curing this infirmity. He further distinguished these "artificiall gifts" as the "arts" practised by the surgeon, for whose benefit Clowes published his treatise.[51] In 1625, Cotta again made the point that the "true artist" or accredited physician received his guidance from God. Both of these writers laid claim by their language, not only to the mystique of the artist, but they have also co-opted the Divine to establish their legitimacy in the treatment of illness.[52]

In 1622, Richard Banister quoted Ecclesiasticus 38:4 on the title page of his treatise in order to substantiate the practitioner's right to attempt a cure: "God hath created medicines of the earth, and he that is wise, will not condemn them."[53] This passage, however, could work in favour of popular or traditional medicine as well as that practised by physicians. But in two medical treatises which appeared in 1651, the full weight of the biblical passage was added when Ecclesiasticus 38: 1, 2 and 4 were given as a reference to justify the use of a physician when illness occurred. One author, the eminent physician and surgeon Alexander Read, quoted the passage on his title page:

Honour the Physician with that honour that is due unto him because of Necessity: for the Lord hath created him. For of the most High cometh healing... The Lord hath created medicines, etc.[54]

Read propounded a non-fatalistic view of illness which argued that although God sent illness, He also provided the means for a cure; this made it incumbent upon the sufferer to try and regain his health.[55] In 1651 Thomas Brugis used the same passage of scripture; his exegesis concluded that the physician (whom he described as "God's Hand") was only marginally less important than God Himself in the treatment of illness.[56] The same biblical quotation reappeared on Peter Leven's title page a few years later coupled with the cryptic admonition "Give unto the Physician, that unto him belongeth."[57] Also relevant is an anonymous seventeenth-century commonplace book of medical quotations and anatomical notes almost certainly written by a professional. One of the first statements in the volume is:

The short life of our Saviour, whilst he was here upon Earth, was, as it were, as spiritual caring, and healing of the Soul, and afterwards of the Body also: such physitians afterwards were his apostles.[58]

This writer's hostility towards popular practitioners was fully documented on the following page:

every one striveth to be a physitian in the Country, no sooner can any one be pricked with a pin, or stung with a Bee, but every one gives his counsel and presenteth himself to be a phisitian for the patient.

The defensive tone of these authors is clear. Indeed, their desperation to secure a scriptural foundation for their work in treating illness can be seen by the fact that Ecclesiasticus 38 is not even in the standard King James version of the Bible. The physicians had to go to the Douay or Jerusalem Bible for it.[59] These are clear indications that many physicians were finding it difficult to maintain a foothold in a society which placed a higher value on spiritual health than physical soundness. Most people chose to leave the latter to more readily available traditional practitioners who charged more reasonable fees for their services, especially when the end result was in the hands of a Higher Power.

Despite the physicians' claims that they were ordained by God for the healing of human illness and despite the weight of historical literature devoted to recording the rise of professional medicine in the seventeenth century, the older concepts were still alive at the end of he century. George Stanhope D.D., Chaplain-in-ordinary to the king, expressed views in the 1690s which were essentially the same as those held early in the century. His *Meditations and Prayers for Sick Persons* leaves no impression that physicians had any role in the treatment of ill health. Stanhope's "Prayer for Sickness" read:

Sanctifie I beseech Thee, this thy Fatherly correction to me and grant that I may receive it with all the Patience and Submission of a Dutifull Child.[60]

In a climate where an all-powerful and righteous God held sway, the costly treatments of licensed practitioners were unnecessary if God willed recovery and a needless waste if the patient died.[61]

Chapter IV
Professional and Lay Medicine: Treatment and Practice

Although the medical profession laid claim to a corpus of medical knowledge which it deemed inaccessible to those lacking the formal education in the classics and humanities offered by the universities, or, in the case of surgeons, the expertise derived from a lengthy apprenticeship, evidence points to the fact that in reality there was no clearly defined separation between the methods used by authorized practitioners and those used by lay or popular practitioners in the treatment of illness. Doctors' records from the period illustrate the striking similarity between their treatments and those used by lay practitioners, including those which were drawn from an oral tradition and handed down from generation to generation.

This homogeneity of method was assisted by members of the professions who wrote for their fellow physicians and surgeons, as well as by those professionals advocating demonopolization of medical knowledge and who aimed at a purely lay readership. A further weakening of the doctors' claims occurred with the airing of the internal dispute between the chemical physicians who adopted the views of Paracelsus and his disciple Van Helmont, and the traditional practitioners of Galenic medicine. In addition, non-professionals published treatises which cited receipts for "cures" by both doctors and lay practitioners.

Dr. John Hall was a university-trained physician who used the treatments commonly associated with Galenic medicine: laxatives, enemas, emetics and bleeding, although he appeared to use phlebotomy or bleeding much less frequently than other forms of removing unhealthy "humours" from his suffering patients.[1] Hall's prescriptions were commonly concoctions of readily available herbs, roots and spices. When Mr. Drayton, a poet, was suffering from a Tertian ague, Hall gave him an "emetick infusion mixed with syrup of violets" which, Hall noted, worked "very well both upwards and downwards."[2] He treated Mrs. Chandler, who was ill with child-bed fever, with a mixture of hartshorn, spring water, syrup of lemons, rosewater, sugar and syrup of red poppies, which he claimed cured her.[3] The young son of a minister who Hall diagnosed as suffering from "Falling sickness," was treated by having "round pieces" of peony root hung about his neck, as well as a sponge soaked in vinegar and rue, applied to his nostrils.[4] The medieval practice of hanging peony root around children's necks as a preventive measure against convulsions was also noted in Lady Sedley's receipt book (1686) and credited to a Dr. Lyons, again demonstrating the amorphous nature of medical "knowledge."[5] The practice was recommended in medical literature as late as 1739, and may have originated with Dioscorides who advised hanging the peony plant "about one" to avoid poisons, bewitchings, fears and devils as well as fevers and agues.[6]

Hall gave a fifty-year-old woman who was bleeding from the mouth a mixture which contained syrup of poppies, rosewater, conserve of roses, bloodstone and sealed earth.[7] To treat a man who had not voided for three days, Hall prescribed a mixture of winter cherry berries, parsley seed, milk, syrup of marshmallows and Holland powder followed by local applications of hot onion and garlic fried in butter and vinegar; the latter treatment "procured urine within an hour, with some stone and gravel."[8] An "electuary" made of finely chopped dates mixed with purified honey cured Mrs. Harvey, five weeks post-partum, of excessive vaginal discharge, pain and weakness in her back.[9] Although Hall has been credited with combining "medical procedures and herbal decoctions with an enlightened cure for scurvy," his prescriptions for scurvy which contained scurvy-grass, water cress and brook-lime were basically the same as or inferior to those used by lay practitioners, many of which also contained oranges and lemons.[10] For example, Lady Sedley's receipt book contained five prescriptions for scurvy: one of these was credited to the renowned anatomist, Richard Lower. But one recipe containing lemons, and one from a layman containing orange juice, were far superior to Dr. Lower's, as well as to Dr. Hall's receipts.[11] Susanna Avery's receipt book (inscribed 1688), contained "A Drinke for the Scurvy" which called for oranges, among other ingredients.[12] In his treatise on diseases of the eye, Richard Banister mentioned a woman who was "famous for curing the Scorby." She administered a drink made from brook-lime and water cresses, "nine times daily." This unknown woman, then, was using a herbal treatment (which is now known to be high in the content of vitamin "C" and specific for the treatment of scurvy) many years before Hall's records were published.[13]

John Symcotts was another university-trained and fully qualified practitioner whose treatments combined elements of folk medicine, superstition, and Galenic tradition. In 1648 he treated the youngest son of the Earl of Bridgewater who had apparently suffered a stroke. A partial list of his efforts to save the unconscious young man's life included blowing tobacco up his nostrils (as well as sneezing powder), warm applications to his head, striking his hands and feet "mightily," inserting mustard and vinegar in his mouth, enemas, suppositories, cupping, scarification, applying plasters and dead pigeons to his feet, holding a hot frying pan close to his head and applying leeches to his rectum. Despite (or more probably because of) Symcotts' efforts, the young man died.[14] Among Symcotts' recipes were two which Symcotts acknowledged as recipts from lay people; one was a prescription for a salve for a "spleen plaster," the other a list of ingredients for a remedy against the plague or the ague which Symcotts ascribed to "Mrs. Rolt of Pertenhall."[15] The latter contained no less than twenty roots, plants or herbs in a base of white wine. When this recipe used by Dr. Symcotts is compared with a recipe found in a seventeenth-century manuscript from the Dorset region which was based on orally transmitted traditions, the Dorset recipe known as "Mrs. Hodges cordiall Water, useful for agues or any infectious diseases," duplicates Symcotts' (or Mrs. Rolt's) recipe almost ingredient for ingredient.[16] Further research is needed to establish firmly the debt which seventeenth-century physicians owed to lay practitioners of earlier generations, but again, the generalization can be made that licensed practitioners could offer no guarantee of cures which were the exclusive property of the professionals.

Symcotts' records offer a further illustration of the blurring of the line between popular and "learned" medicine. In 1635 when Dr. Symcotts was suffering from gout, his brother, a London merchant, wrote to suggest that his brother try the treatment by which he had cured himself the previous year; this "cure" consisted of a paste made from yeast, egg white and alum which was spread on brown paper and bound about the foot.[17] The editors of Symcotts' case records cite the latter as a striking commentary on the state of seventeenth-century medicine. But it is an excellent example of how contemporary lay people perceived the limited capacity of the medical profession, even to the extent of their inability to treat themselves effectively.

The notes of an unknown doctor who lived and worked in the North Riding of Yorkshire in the early seventeenth century, while not as extensive as Hall's and Symcotts' records, show that purges and vomits were the mainstay of his practice and that his medicines were usually made from "simple and conservative" ingredients such as senna.[18]

The analysis of 83 medical treatises which were published between 1640 and 1660, reveals that while 39 were ostensibly intended for use by the professionals, only 9 were written in Greek or Latin, thus placing them out of the reach of all but the formally educated. A further 10 publications were directed to lay as well as professional use.[19] Thus, of the literature for licensed physicians and surgeons, some 40 treatises offered "cures" which could be easily duplicated by lay persons (indeed in some cases, cures or treatments were ascribed to lay practitioners). The remaining 30 odd treatises were clearly intended for lay use.

Ralph Williams, "practitioner in Physick and Chyrurgerie," stated that he wrote for the professions; he described treatments for plague, tertian fevers and gout, all based on herbs, roots, bark or other readily available ingredients.[20] Williams included Galen's cure for gout: old cheese soaked in the broth of a gammon of bacon and made into a plaster for local application.[21] Robert Bayfield of Norwich also wrote for the professions, especially "to help young and greene students in Physick and Chyrurgery."[22] His prescription for various cordials to treat the plague are made up of readily available materials such as root of angelica, wormwood vine, conserve of roses, treacle and mithridate.[23] For inflammation of the breast, Bayfield prescribed the same concoction as for stomach ache with vomiting: syrup of roses, syrup of rhubarb and senna.[24]

Three Fellows of the College of Physicians in London published a scholarly work in 1650: *A Treatise of the Rickets Being a Disease Common to Children.*[25] The authors, headed by the highly respected Francis Glisson, left no doubt that their work, which has been described by twentieth-century medical historians as "a magnificent work of clinical and pathological observation," was intended for the benefit of professional practitioners.[26] The treatment of rickets which they outlined, however, offered nothing new or original that lay beyond the compass of traditional or popular medicine. Their research undoubtedly assisted lay practitioners in the diagnosis of rickets, while the treatments which they recommended were customarily non-specific, described by the doctors as simples and compounds *"readily available* in shops such as rue, spica roots, Fernbrake, betony, Fennell, caraway, dill."[27] The regimen, typically Galenical, included an initial preparation of the passages with enemas, vomits and purges, and finally, external applications of camomile, marigold and earthworms, as well as ointments made of herbs, butter and nutmeg.[28] Glisson and his colleagues failed to make any connection between their clinical discoveries, which related to diagnosis and description, and their treatment of the disease; in the case of rickets, it was pointless to seek the help of licensed physicians. Indeed, in one medical compendium published by a lay person for non-professionals, a receipt which contained the specific treatment for rickets appeared in 1655.[29]

Examples of works directed to both professional and lay audiences were those by Robert Pemel and Martin Blockwich.[30] Nicholas Culpeper was the most prolific and outstanding representative of the group who wrote for the lay person. There were, however, other licensed practitioners who wrote specifically for the benefit of lay practitioners and for those who for various reasons were interested in self-treatment.[31] John Tanner's

The Hidden Treasures of the Art of Physick and James Cooke's treatise
on surgery, were typical of the publications which like Culpeper's were
directed at laymen.[32]

Aside from the books whose authors were clearly identified with
the medical profession in one way or another, other compendia were
published for the benefit of the lay practitioner or to give directions
for self-treatment. The most ambitious of these was published in 1655
under the pseudonym "Philiatros" and purported to contain one
thousand seven hundred and twenty "Receipts fitted for the cure of all
sorts of Infirmities whether Internal or External, Acute or Chronical
that are incident to the body of Man."[33] The "receipts" were contributed
or approved by a variety of persons and provide an interesting commentary
not only on the minimal control exercised by the universities and the
doctors in the dissemination of medical knowledge, but also on the way
that a prescription from a lay person was perceived as having as much
merit as one from a licensed practitioner. Contributors include 22 doctors,
41 males from either the aristocracy or gentry, 13 women with the title
of Countess or lady, 32 women with the designation "Mrs.", one good
wife and two women without any designation; the heaviest contributor
was a Mrs. Downing, with 16 prescriptions. In this publication, then,
the contributions of lay practitioners outnumbered those by doctors by
four to one.

In the same year, W.M., who claimed to have been a former servant
of the Queen, published *The Queen's Closet opened,* a book which proved
so popular, subsequent editions appeared in 1671, 1674, 1683 and 1698.[34]
One possible reason for the book's popularity was the author's claim
that the queen had actually used many of the prescriptions. Listed among
the contributors of receipts to the "Queen's closet" were 29 physicians
and surgeons, 15 men with titles or from the gentry, 16 countesses and
ladies, 1 bishop and only 3 from what could be considered the lower
classes.[35]

Moreover, there appears to be no distinction between the illnesses
for which the physician offered receipts and those for which lay persons
offered their favoured cures. Philiatros published two cures for the gout
which were attributed to Mr. Peacock and Mr. John Cornwallis, as well
as five or six treatments by unnamed contributors.[36] Of the latter, one
was designated, the "best" cure for gout; it contained black soap and
the yolks of raw eggs bound to the afflicted part by a plaster of egg
whites and flour.[37] W.M.'s treatise offered "Dr. Stevens' cure for gout,"
made up of his famous "water," plus sheep's suet, boar's grease, wax
and "neet's foot oyl"; a prescription for gout by a lay person contained
sheep's suet and wax, as well as herbs while another unnamed contributor
included the "neet's foot oil" favoured by Dr. Stevens.[38] Lady Oxford's
"Oyl of Excester" was described as a cure for gout and sciatica. It contained

olive oil plus seventeen herbs, plants and flowers. Mr. Peacock's cure, while more modest in content, also contained flowers and leaves.[39] It can be seen, therefore, that there was no great distinction between the ingredients used by professionals and lay practitioners.

In some instances, receipts by lay persons were of a high quality. Both of the 1655 treatises contained prescriptions for scurvy which were high in vitamin C content.[40] The receipt for the cure of rickets in children was far superior to anything offered by Dr. Glisson and his confreres in their scholarly treatise; copious amounts of milk were recommended over an extended length of time, a treatment which subsequent research has proven to be specific for the prevention of rickets.[41] Each of the books contained receipts with elements of superstition such as the method for curing a wound at a distance (by washing a cloth stained in blood from the wound) or writing the letters AOGL in blood above the wound.[42] W.M. and Philiatros both offered the following "cure" for the plague: hold a chicken, whose rump has been plucked, to the plague sore so that it draws out the poison with its beak. When it dies, apply another fowl and continue to do so until the birds no longer die.[43] This curious treatment reappeared eleven years later in the pamphlet *Certain Necessary Directions as well for the Cure of the Plague and for the Prevention of Infection,* which was issued by the College of Physicians.[44] This illustrates how the most prestigious professionals, representing the medical elite, "borrowed" from lay tradition and practice, especially when they were dealing with illnesses for which their own treatments had proved singularly ineffectual.[45]

There were other publications which combined varying degrees of the occult with medical practice, such as Samuel Boulton's *Medicina, Magica Tamen Physica.* Boulton propounded a bizarre theory which claimed that the "excrements of living creatures," retained some of the "vital spirits." He suggested various ways in which animal excrement could be used. For example, dog's excrement was good for curing diseases of the throat and palate, according to Boulton.[46] In 1658, John Schroder, doctor of Physic, published a book describing how various animals, birds, fish and insects could be used in treating disease.[47] The ideas presented by these authors can probably be traced to the work of the classical herbalist Dioscorides, who included sections on the use of dung and urine (human and animal) as well as various animal parts. Brockbank has shown how heavily the London Pharmacopoeia, the official publication of the College of Physicians, drew upon Dioscorides' work.[48] Even practitioners of learning and repute such as Thomas Sydenham and Thomas Willis were advocating the use of animal products, including excreta, late in the seventeenth century.[49]

A recent paper has noted the peculiar ability of seventeenth-century minds to live in two worlds, citing the presence of occult and antioccult tendencies in Kepler, Bacon and Newton. John Locke and Robert Boyle shared Newton's surreptitious interest in alchemy under a cloak of sworn secrecy while Kepler's interest in astrology and mysticism led him to the use of horoscopes to explain his own illness. A study of the occult tradition in the English university has stressed the impossibility of eliminating "scholastic and magical modes of thought" from the "scientific revolution."[50] Not surprisingly, elements of magic and superstition existed in receipts, such as those given in the medical compendia for staunching blood. The same elements, however, can also be found in the writings of Willis, whose work as an neuroanatomist has been highly praised. For example, he suggested the following cure for jaundice:

Take the fresh urine of a person made at one time, with ashes of the ash tree as much as suffices to reduce to a paste which may be formed into three equal balls to be placed near a hearth or stove. As these dry and harden the jaundice will vanish.[51]

Willis went on to say that he found this cure effective when other remedies had failed; also revealing was his comment that the treatment was "very familiar to the vulgar." In other words Willis did not hesitate to appropriate and endorse treatments associated with the sphere of popular medicine, particularly when other standard medical treatments of the day had failed to produce a cure.

When the chemical or Helmontian physicians attacked the traditional Galenical school of medicine to which most physicians and surgeons subscribed, a further weakening of the doctors' claims to a body of knowledge which lay beyond the comprehension of the uneducated occurred. This group of doctors rejected the humoral theory of illness for one formulated by Paracelsus in which the preservation of the "vital spirits" was foremost.[52] Although the radicals claimed that they treated their patients conservatively without the depletion of their body fluids (or spirits), by phlebotomy, vomits and purges, in practice their treatments retained a remarkable similarity to those carried out by the Galenical school.[53] Moreover, their polemical attacks on the majority of the profession only served to damage the credibility of the medical profession as a whole.

Thomas O'Dowd, a leading proponent of the new method, described his "cures" which were produced by administering chemical medicine; one "cure" which he took the credit for resulted in 45 vomits and more than 50 stools, while another patient who took less than a grain of O'Dowd's medicine "fell to vomit and stool without intermission."[54] Chemical physicians such as George Thomson and George Starkey levelled blistering attacks at the establishment practitioners. Thomson, a fully accredited physician and apologist for chemical medicine, documented the case of a woman whose vital spirits had been disturbed with the result that three large "stones" had formed in her colon. Thomson's treatment was to administer "emeto-diaphoreticks and emeto-catharticks," a treatment which not only directly contradicted the title of his treatise, but was essentially the same as Galenical medicine.[55]

Starkey, a proponent of the chemical method, levelled a blistering attack on the Galenists in 1656 in which he commented on the doctors' appropriation of folk or popular medicine and the way they had corrupted it to serve their own ends:

...but whatever they [Galenists] have that may do good, they have it from the accidental experiments of old wives, and good folks, who have found or known much good done by this or that Herb or Simple...then when Doctors after had drawn it into Receipts.[56]

Starkey also contended that in many cases people living in villages who did not have access to a doctor, and poor people who could not afford one, often cured themselves by simple methods and at less risk than if a doctor was involved.[57] Thus Starkey established the legitimacy of popular medicine vis-a-vis Galenical or professional medicine. What he failed to acknowledge was the fact that many chemical physicians still clung to Galenical remedies although claiming a different theoretical base.[58] Moreover, as late as 1679, one "chemical" doctor was advocating "oyl and spirits of cinnamon" for illnesses involving the heart and head and especially for shortness of breath, "oyl of cloves" for wounds, yellow jaundice and haemorrhoids, "oyl of nutmegs" for "cholick and indispositions of the liver," all treatments well within the range of folk or traditional medicine.[59]

Another important mid-century critic of the medical profession, Noah Biggs, appeared to criticize the content and method of medical education and practice (as well as the organization of the universities), with a view to promoting the chemical method.[60] Like Starkey, he harkened to the traditional methods of treatment which simple folk employed. In so doing, however, he was not advocating a retreat to the past, but arguing for a more progressive medical tradition which would use better experimental methods, employ anatomical studies, expand its knowledge of herbs and explore the new realm of chemical medicine. Biggs based his arguments for reform on his observations of an impotent and ineffectual medical profession who were taught to "mouth out the perfection of their Art" even though they knew from their lack of success that they were only "catching at painted Butterflies."[61]

Throughout the seventeenth century, doctors and laymen both looked to astrology as a tool to assist in the diagnosis and prognosis of illness. Astrology was one of Culpeper's interests and he published some of his theories regarding astrology and illness in 1651.[62] Dr. Richard Foster, a member of the College of Physicians in London (and its president in 1601-1604 and again in 1615) was one of the few members of this august group who made a study of astronomy and astrology as an adjunct to the study of medicine.[63] For the most part, however, astrology remained the preoccupation of a fringe group of self-taught practitioners such as Simon Forman and Elias Ashmole, both of whom dabbled in the occult, as well as of the large number of people seeking information helpful in self-treatment.

At the turn of the century, the notorious astrologer Simon Forman had already battled the doctors for almost two decades over his unlicensed treatment of the sick and crippled by the use of magic and astrology.[64] A few years later, Richard Napier offered a combination of orthodox treatment, astrological diagnosis and spiritual counselling in his very successful practice. [65] In 1651, Ashmole had good results when he treated himself using a method suggested by an "astroligian" after previous treatment by a licensed physician, Dr. Wharton, had failed.[66] Ashmole had begun the study of physick in 1650, and his efforts encompassed a wide variety of subjects in addition to magic and astrology. In 1657, his pursuit of knowledge led him on a journey to visit an eclectic group of practitioners which included a botanist, a physician (an "ingenious man"), an apothecary, and a female practitioner.[67]

A number of publications appeared which encouraged self-diagnosis and treatment by the use of astrological signs and charts. One of these by R. Turner was published in 1655.[68] It was dedicated to "Doctor Trigge, Doctor in Physick." Such an acknowledgment of the cobbler-doctor who had gained fame through his successful treatment of large numbers of sufferers, could only serve to strengthen the tie between astrology, the occult and popular medicine.[69] Genevieve Miller has commented on the fact that astrological theories exerted a powerful influence "on the mind of the average person" and the way in which medical compendia were a mixture of Galenic and astrological theories.[70] Hugh Dick's study demonstrated that astrology was practised widely throughout the seventeenth century, often as a "cloak to furtive medical activity." Dick's conclusion in this regard supports the position that astrology aided and abetted the practice of popular medicine.[71] He also points out that the main opposition to astrology came from philosophic and religious influences, rather than from the medical profession, a fact which demonstrates the uncritical attitude of the profession to "fringe" branches of medical practice.[72]

Seventeenth-century almanacs were another medium for the dissemination of medical information. At two pence a copy, one conservative estimate has placed three or four million copies in the hands of seventeenth-century men and women from all walks of life.[73] They offered the usual cures for common ailments supplemented by astrological charts. The best times for bleeding, purging and vomits were demonstrated by the use of astrology in Naworth's "A New Almanack and Prognostication for the yeare of our Lord and Saviour Jesus Christ, 1644."[74] Another almanac for the year 1646 gave a table which determined the different "complexions," (choler, phlegme, melancholy and sanguine) in order to calculate the best times for blood-letting when considered in conjunction with astrological signs.[75] This almanac also offered cures for gout and the King's Evil.[76] Wharton's almanac for 1648 predicted an increase in fevers, coughs and consumption as the result of an impending eclipse.[77] In addition, almanacs afforded a platform for the advertisement of both licensed and unlicensed practitioners.[78]

Bearing in mind the constraints of literacy and their effects on the spread of medical knowledge, the fact that must be acknowledged is that the majority of authors as well as the literate public perceived no distinct line between the "cures" which the doctors touted and those which were used by lay practitioners or between those which had originated in an oral tradition and those which had come out of the so-called Galenical school.[79] Contemporary sources reveal to the twentieth-century historian that the bulk of the doctor's frequently expensive "cures" were no different from those cheaply and readily available to the population at large; moreover, this fact was proclaimed through the printed word by professionals and laymen alike who consciously or unconsciously exposed the falsity of the doctor's claims.

Evidence of the way in which historians have tended to take the physicians' claims at face value can be found in Peter Burke's study of popular culture in early modern Europe. Burke cites Sir Thomas Browne's book as an example of the increased "intellectual content in the age of the scientific revolution." Browne, a prestigious medical practitioner, claimed that his work *Pseudoxia Epidemica* was "a study of received tenets and commonly-presumed truths" about illness. In it he attempted to correct the "erroneous disposition of the people whose uncultivated understandings made them credulous..." The full irony of Burke's choice of Browne's book to illustrate "scientific progress" can only be appreciated by an awareness of the fact that Browne believed in witches. It was his testimony at a trial in 1664 which resulted in two women being convicted and hanged.[80]

Despite their superior academic training (or in the case of surgeons, lengthy apprenticeship), doctors were aware that in many cases, their cures did not work and they were willing, therefore, to borrow from popular practitioners. This is why Willis noted that he tried the folk cure for a jaundice which then was "happily cured although resisting many other remedies." Among other examples of "last resort" cures by popular practitioners was an old woman, described by John Smith, doctor in Physick, who had cured "one that was incurable" by using folk knowledge.[81] Robert Boyle gave the prescription for a cure of "an obstinate Tumour of the knee that had baffled some surgeon"; it consisted of green colewart leaves (with red veins) which were bruised and laid on the affected part.[82] Starkey spoke of old women who cured "deserted patients" or in other words, patients whose doctors had abandoned them after failing to alleviate their problems.[83] It was Starkey also who charged "Even the most serious of them will confess, that all their Art consist in experimental Receipts." Physicians, then, were grasping at straws, or to use Biggs' term, catching at "painted butterflies," a mindset which enabled them to accept the efforts of popular practitioners when they had exhausted the poorly defined body of knowledge which was generally associated with seventeenth-century medical training.

In conclusion, any sharp distinction between "popular" and professional medical practice and treatment in Stuart England appears to be untenable. The concepts of a unique corpus of established, academic knowledge on the one hand, and of a backward, simple folk medicine on the other, are equally misleading. Within the published literature as well as available physicians' and lay records, the two merged together into a largely amorphous whole. The recognition of this fact is vital in assessing the nature and position of popular medicine in this period. In essence, it was neither "fringe" nor "alternative" health care, but an integral part of an unconscious, interdependent "system."[84] Evaluated in these terms, the continued vitality of popular medicine throughout the century was reasonable and, in the main, noncontentious. These points can be fully illustrated by the following case study of the enduring role of lay female practitioners within this society.

Chapter V
Women's Role in Stuart Medicine:
A Case Study of Popular Practitioners

Since most medical historians of the early modern period have written from the perspective of professional medicine, they have either completely ignored the role of ordinary women in the provision of medical services, or dismissed them with patronizing terms such as wise women, herb women, white witches, or simply old women, often implying that they were little better than quacks.[1] The part played by gentlewomen in the treatment of illness, while receiving slightly greater recognition, has been similarly undervalued and glossed over. By contrast, it will be demonstrated that women played a central role in Stuart health care. Because of their gender, women were only very rarely found amongst the ranks of professional surgeons and physicians. As a result, academic studies have focussed on plotting the linear development of the medical profession (and in many instances equating this with improvement in medical practice), thereby ignoring the contribution of women. This marginalization of half the population, however, seriously distorts the entire nature of health care in seventeenth-century England. As a readily identifiable and significant group of non-professional healers in this period, a case study of the role of women sheds considerable light upon the topic of popular medicine.

The normal route into the practice of physic, education in grammar schools and universities, was closed to women. Similarly, women were only rarely apprenticed within surgery guilds. Bishops seldom granted licenses to women who wished to practice physick, as will be seen below, and thus most female practice was not only unlicensed, but unrecorded in the 'normal' documentary sense. The main route into the practice of formal surgery was through the traditional right within all encorporated crafts for widows to carry on the profession of their deceased spouses.[2] This is an important topic which stands in need of intensive archival study. At present, while it is clear that women could in isolated cases enter the medical 'profession' in this manner, just as they could become episcopally licensed physicians, in most cases, for reasons unknown but which must be related to the whole concept of health care and the place of women in it, they do not appear to have normally availed themselves of this privilege. In a study of the barber-surgeons of York, Margaret Barnet noted that the licensing of Isabell Warwicke as a surgeon in 1572 was contingent on her "good behaviour," a restriction which was not imposed upon male surgeons. Similarly, Adrian Colman, widow of surgeon Nicholas Colman of Norwich, was licensed to practice surgery in 1596 with, as Pelling and Webster have pointed out, some nominal restrictions on her practice.[3] Pelling and Webster have not clearly defined what these restrictions were, but there is the implication that Colman's services were available only to those who had been unsuccessfully treated by other practitioners. Although both Colman and Warwicke were apparently experienced and skilful practitioners, the fact that restrictions were imposed on their practices may be a clue to the type of opposition which widows faced in gaining admittance to the practice of surgery, under their traditional right, in the early modern period. By 1641, a tax survey of the London Barber-Surgeons Company showed only a single female member among the 295 identified Company freemen.[4] The Annals of the Barber-Surgeons of London revealed a similarly isolated case, that of "gentleman's daughter" Katharina Bowshy, who became apprenticed to a barber surgeon and his wife in 1660.[5] The same source disclosed a few examples of male barber surgeons' apprentices who were bound to female masters; the wife of barber surgeon Thomas Asbridge continued to supervise her apprentice, Mark Nurse, after her husband's death. Mistress Wooton complained to the company about her apprentice in 1616, while in 1627, the apprentice of Solomon Carr's wife was brought before the authorities. In June 1658, Daniel Alderson was apprenticed to Katherine Alderson.[6] The apprentices' rolls of Bristol for the year 1681 reveal that Margaret Pope took an apprentice, Sarah Sanders, "a yeoman's child," for five years' teaching and instruction "according to her best skill and knowledge in the art and business of Doctress and Chirurgion."[7] In 1651, Sir Gerard Barrington was glowing in his praise of an unnamed female surgeon who took "good and tender care" of his lame leg.[8] Pelling included 37 female practitioners in her study of Norwich for the years 1550-1640, but did not give specific details regarding their background and training although she noted that some of them had "formal qualifications" and "status in official records." For example, noting that part of the group had licences in physick, and surgery, we are not told how many, nor how the licenses were obtained. Similarly, we are not told how many "were involved in apprenticeship."[9] Pelling and Webster have, however, concluded for the sixteenth century that, although the odd woman obtained a license to practice surgery, women generally practiced surgery, especially in the countryside, without a license.[10] There is a strong likelihood that Mrs.

Withers, the bone setter whom Ralph Josselin called in 1660 to set his daughter's arm which had been dislocated (as well as to treat his wife's foot), was one of these skilful, albeit unlicensed practitioners.[11]

Sir George Clark, apologist and historian of the Royal College of Medicine, closed his eyes to the reality of widespread popular medicine as it was practised in the seventeenth century.[12] Due to the very fact that historical work has focussed on the College, all other medical practice has disappeared from view, leaving the twentieth-century reader with the impression that seventeenth-century London was well served by a small group of "modern," stalwart doctors, well-intentioned, well-trained and all male. Another study devoted to the profession demonstrated that some 814 doctors ministered to the health needs of the provinces in the years 1603-1640, moving its author to conclude: "Therefore instead of having no care, or at best care by quacks or charlatans, they had well-trained doctors by their standards."[13] Not only has the author of this study, J. Raach, labelled all other alternative types of medicine and practitioners as dangerous and unethical, a position which is untenable given the homogeneity of treatment practised by lay and professionals alike, he has ignored the whole problem of demography and distribution which his own study demonstrates.[14] In the light of the foregoing, Raach's statement seems overly optimistic at best and grossly inaccurate at its worst. Even so, a more serious flaw is Raach's inclusion in his study of only two women practitioners in the provinces. One of these, Katherine Green, practised in Royston, Herefordshire, around 1626 under the authority of a bishop's license.[15] But it is the other woman, Prudence Potter, whose presence in the study calls attention to the deficiencies in Raach's work.

Prudence Potter lived and practised in Devonshire until her death in 1689 at the age of seventy-seven. The inscription on her tombstone spoke of her skill as a physician, surgeon and midwife.[16] Raach included her name among his 814 practitioners on the basis of a local study which was one of only two which he used in compiling his roster.[17] An examination of Raach's "doctors" for the county of Devonshire illustrates the methodological problems associated with the only detailed study of medical practitioners outside of London. He included 58 individuals: 24 with some form of university degree, 24 with bishop's licenses, 5 names from the Prerogative Court of Canterbury, Principle Probate Registry London, one name from a visitation list and 4 names were from the aforementioned study. For these four practitioners (including Prudence Potter) no license or qualification is shown; Raach apparently accepted the perception of local contemporaries that the four were competent and active medical practitioners. Thus, in going beyond his own self-imposed criteria as to what constituted a qualified physician in provincial England, Raach has pointed out both the limitations and the inconsistencies of his study. If only one local study revealed that one of four active, assumedly competent (albeit unlicensed) practitioners was a woman, it is not inconceivable that when local studies for all of the counties have been completed, they will disclose a significant number of women who were skilled and respected practitioners. In fact the only existing detailed analysis of all medical practitioners within a specific locality, completed by Margaret Pelling for Norwich, has demonstrated precisely this. By Pelling's use of an "extended range of sources," instead of relying solely on official documentation, as is customary in occupational analysis, she has reclaimed women, a minority group of great importance in Stuart health care.[18]

All of Raach's main sources of information almost automatically excluded women, due to the social and cultural characteristics of this period. Barred from institutions of higher education, unlikely to be issued (or to require) formal licenses to practice, women also, in comparison to men, left less documentary evidence of their occupations in general. Married women as a rule did not produce wills, and single women were more likely to identify themselves in these documents in terms of their marital status (widow, spinster) than by occupation. A further example of the unconscious bias in a study such as that composed by Raach can be derived simply from the differences of gender designations within correspondence. For example, Raach includes a "Dr." Bauer whose legitimacy is accepted solely on the basis of being so designated in a contemporary letter although there is no evidence of educational qualifications, license, will, or even a first name. Raach, however, has failed to include female practitioners mentioned in diaries and letters, but whose names, by tradition, were not dignified by the title "doctor."[19] In brief, a methodologically unsound study cannot be expected to provide an accurate portrayal of medical practice; in the case of women, this is even more apparent.

R.S. Roberts has also presented a picture of an exclusively male medical service operating in the provinces in his study "The Personnel and Practice of Medicine in Tudor and Stuart England." Roberts' presentation is slanted toward the professionals as a whole, a fact demonstrated by only two allusions, in passing, to "wise country *people*" and "local wise *people*" (emphasis mine); by such terminology, he has subtly deprived rural women of even a token acknowledgement of their traditional place in medical practice.[20]

Leading social and intellectual authorities on seventeenth-century England, for example, Christopher Hill and Charles Webster, have also perpetuated the neglect of women practitioners and treated them in a peremptory manner. Hill refers to "the white witch, the cunning man or woman of whom there was one in most villages" as the main alternative resource of people who lacked access to licensed practitioners. Having thus defined the importance of this group, Hill omits any further reference to women practitioners of the lower class in his lengthy discussion of seventeenth-century medicine; he makes no mention at all of the large number of gentlewomen who practiced the healing arts.[21]

In his 1975 study, Charles Webster devoted one paragraph to women practitioners in which most of his attention was directed to gentlewomen. He mentions Elizabeth Ray, a blacksmith's wife, as an example of lower-class women who practiced medicine, as well as the usual unnamed "herb women."[22] Webster, however, failed to enlarge on the existence of these shadowy figures until his more recent work which he published in conjunction with Margaret Pelling whose research has revealed the substantial number of female medical practitioners in sixteenth and early seventeenth-century Norwich. Pelling's and Webster's conclusions for the sixteenth-century (as well as Pelling's up to 1640) have demonstrated the widespread and influential role of traditional medicine which remained independent of the small group of medical graduates headed by a "university-educated elite."[23]

The group of female practitioners who have been given token acknowledgement in the history of medicine is that which was drawn from the ranks of gentlewomen who ministered to the health needs of families, friends and neighbours. Even here, some distortion of the role which these women played can be found in the work of previous generations of medical historians such as that of Leonard Guthrie. Guthrie adopted the perspective of the medical profession and gave credit to the profession rather than oral and traditional sources (including herbals) for much of the skill and knowledge which these ladies possessed.[24] This interpretation, as will be seen, is at odds with evidence from seventeenth-century diaries, manuscripts and "recipe" books. A further denigration of women's contribution has occurred at the hands of historians such as Antonia Fraser who has chosen to call their work "nursing" although it is clear that most women practitioners acted without the supervision of a doctor and provided exactly the same type of treatment, in many cases, as a doctor.[25]

Since gentlewomen and ladies have left more written records of their work than women from the lower classes, more attention has been paid to them, a situation which more studies like that of Pelling will serve to redress. But whether one places these privileged women to the fore, or, (like Hill), the country "wise women," sufficient recognition has not been given to the important part which women played in...health care and medical treatment in seventeenth-century England.

Municipal records have yielded examples of female practitioners of humble origins whose status, although unofficial, was confirmed by local records such as the account books of boroughs and parishes: Widow Foote who received 20 shillings from the corporation of Worchester in

1651 to cure Widow Hutchins' lame leg; Goodwife Wells of Cowden had ten shillings for "curing" the hand of Elizabeth Skinner; Mary Olyve of Mayfield, Sussex, was paid six shillings and eight pence for curing a lame boy; widow Thurston of Cratfield was paid 15 shillings in 1640 by the church warden for healing a boy, while Johane Shorley of Somerset received £5 as partial payment for curing Thomas Dudderidge in 1653 (with more promised when the cure was complete).[26]

After their marriage in 1615, Alice and Lawrence Wright became joint keepers of the Lazar house at St. Bennet's gates in Norwich. Following Lawrence's death, Alice became responsible for the medical treatment of the inmates. For this she was paid, under contract to the city, between 15 shillings and one pound per case. She was succeeded by the Stephensons, a man and wife, with Rose Stephenson assuming the responsibilities of medical care, including the treatment of scurvy and scald head.[27] The treatment of scald head was one of the conditions where women had apparently acquired some expertise. For example, in the "Regulations for government of St. Bartholomew's Hospital" which were set forth in 1656, provision was made for the hiring of two physicians, and an apothecary, two surgeons and a woman "to cure scald heads and leprosy at from 20s to 40s the cure."[28]

The assize records for Sussex in the year 1622 yield a less fortituous example of a woman practitioner: in 1622 when Elizabeth Merriall wanted to treat her ailing husband, she consulted Mercy Duplake, possibly the local wise woman in Mayfield, Sussex. On her advice, Elizabeth purchased a penny's worth of 'sparmaceti' (or so she thought) from the mercer, one Francis Parkhurst. Unfortunately, Francis became confused and gave Mrs. Merriall mercury instead of sparmaceti. As a result, the patient died.[29]

In addition to the foregoing "official" sources, recorded "cures" which bear women's names are "unofficial" sources which not only confirm the existence of women healers, but often suggest the social profiles of ordinary women. In this category fall several seventeenth-century folk remedies from the Dorset region: "Goody Wilsheirs, a receipt for a woman that cannot be delivered," "my sister Elizabeth's receit very choice against a consumption," "Mrs. Hodges cordiall water."[30] Further examples of women whose names were associated with prescriptions or "cures" are Anne Kirby, Goodwife Veazy, Widow Scott, Goodwife Worsted and "the old lady of Oxford."[31] In addition, there are anonymous women whose cures were recorded, but not their names. John Symcotts, physician in the provinces, described a cure by an unnamed woman who successfully treated a woman stricken with a palsy. He also described (and used) a cure which was suggested by a beggar woman.[32] The Verney memoirs yield the "dreadful old woman" whose ointment was recommended for treating Sir Ralph Verney's leg.[33]

In contrast to the paucity of evidence regarding women of the lower classes who were actively engaged in the practice of popular medicine, diaries and letters of the period abound in references to the skilled group of unofficial practitioners who were women of gentle or noble birth. In her diary, which she began at the end of the sixteenth-century, Lady Hoby repeatedly referred to her practice in physick as well as surgery, which she carried out at home and in the neighbouring parish. Much of her time was occupied in dressing sores and wounds, some of which she dressed twice a day. For example from February 4 to February 18, 1600, she dressed a minimum of two patients daily, often attending them twice a day.[34] On one occasion she treated a servant who had cut his foot with a hatchet and at another time a servant with a badly cut hand.[35] Not only did Lady Margaret consult an herbal, she enjoyed reading medical and metaphysical works such as Timothie Bright's *A Treatise of Melancholie*.[36] Skilled in the preparation of remedies, she sent a purgative mixture which she had made to her cousin's ailing servant; on another occasion she "made a salve for a sore breast." In 1604 she visited a woman who was mute because of an apparent mental disorder but she evidently was unsuccessful in getting the patient to talk.[37] Similarly, when Lady Anne Clifford's mother was ill and in "sore danger of death" in 1616, Anne sent cordials and conserves to aid her recovery. Anne's actions were particularly appropriate since her mother had enjoyed a reputation as a skilful healer and had passed on her expertise and knowledge to her daughter.[38] Anne's aunt, Lady Warwick, shared her sister's skill and sent plague medicine to Anne and her mother when they were exposed to the plague in 1603.[39]

Gentlewoman Alice Thornton also credited her mother with having great skill in healing "notwithstanding all the meanes of physicians or others."[40] Alice shared her mother's knowledge and experienced success in treating patients such as the man with a "cutt hand which was lame," as well as her own ailments.[41] She credited a remedy containing muskedine, which she got from a friend, 'Madame Grahme,' for restoring her health and strength when Dr. Wittie, a physician, failed to help.[42] Like Lady Clifford, Alice treated her mother in her terminal illness using home treatments such as "bagges with fried oates, butter and camomell chopt, layed to her sides."[43] From Alice's description, her mother probably died of pneumonia, in which case Alice's home remedy was a reasonable one, given the limits of medical knowledge of the day.

Various female members of the Barrington family supplied other family members with medications and treatments. When her mother was suffering from gout, Mary Gerard sent her some "oyl of Exeter," while sometime later, she sent a salve which was instrumental in greatly improving Lady Barrington's health.[44] In turn, Lady Barrington, who was highly regarded for her knowledge and skill in medicine, was consulted for advice on the treatment of sick children on at least three occasions.[45] She also received a request for a prescription for sore eyes which was known as "Sister Evarards prescription for sore eyes."[46]

When Brilliana Harley's son Edward was living in Oxford and attending university in 1639, his mother continued to assume responsibility for his health, sending medicine and advice such as "bessor stone" and "2 grains of orampotably" to be taken in 2 spoonsful of "cordius watter."[47] In May of the same year she suggested he should drink some "scurvy gras pounded and strained" with beer in order to purge his blood.[48] When Edward had sore eyes, Mrs. Wilkinson, the wife of the headmaster, treated him. Brilliana sent this message to Mrs. Wilkinson: "I thank Mrs. W. for her care of it in which she supplied my place."[49] Lady Harley sent a piece of angelica root to Edward, instructing him to carry it in his pocket and eat it periodically as a means of promoting health.[50] That Lady Harley saw nothing amiss in continuing to treat her son who was residing at a major university centre which was particularly well-supplied with physicians can be taken as a measure of the high level of confidence which gentlewomen enjoyed in medical matters, or conversely for the relative low esteem in which professionals were held.[51]

Lady Anne Howard, Countess of Arundel, (1595-1630) was famous for her skill and knowledge of medicine; her work has been described by her biographer:

all kind of people who either wanting will, or means to go to doctors and chirurgeons, come to her for the curing of their wounds and distempers. And her charity herein was so famous that not only neighbours, but several out of other shires, twenty, forty and more miles distant did resort unto her to that end, and scarce a day passed in which many did not come, sometimes more than three score have been counted in one day.... She ordered divers kinds of drugs to be brought every year to make her salves and medicines, and herself in person would be present at the making of them to see and be more sure they should be well done and good.[52]

During the Civil War, Lady Ann Halkett wrote of treating "three score" wounded soldiers using her own "plaisters and balsom." One of the soldiers had a particularly severe head wound which exposed his brain but Lady Halkett carefully dressed him and he recovered, a testimony to the lady's intrepid spirit as well as her great skill.[53] On another occasion, Lady Halkett's knowledge enabled her to save her own life by directing a servant to prepare "cordialls" which she herself was too ill to prepare.[54] Lucy Hutchinson's memoirs describe how a gentlewoman successfully treated five wounded men, some of them with "dangerous" injuries, with "excellent balsams and plaster in her closet."[55]

Lady Warwick (1625-1678) sent all the remedies she could think of when one of her husband's servants was gravely ill; she also sent a "palsy balsam" to a woman rendered speechless by the palsy.[56] Lady Warwick's sister, Lady Ranelagh, left a manuscript of "My Lady Ranelagh's Choice Receipts." Undated, it contains some prescriptions attributed to Lady Warwick, suggesting "the possibility that Lady Warwick collaborated with her sister in its production."[57] The wife of the Warwicks' chaplain, Mrs. Elizabeth Walker, was also an outstanding female practitioner who had through industry, labour and experience acquired great skill as both a surgeon and physician. She kept a great store of "vomits, purges, sudorifics, cordials, pectorals...syrups, strong waters," on hand and studied English medical books.[58]

The pages of Dr. John Symotts' case book disclosed the names of at least eleven titled women as well as five gentlewomen (including his sister) who were engaged in medical activities at the popular level.[59] Further examples of well-born women who shared this interest in popular medicine include Lady Margaret Oxinden of Deane who sent an ointment and cordial for the relief of her terminally ill niece, Ann Oxinden. She promised "...I will make her a tisan to-morrow and send her to eas the paynfulness of her cof."[60] In 1627, Thomas Meautys sent "some of that syropp of ella campana" which his sister had made to Lady Jane Bacon noting that he and his friends had derived much benefit from it; he also sent the receipt for making it.[61] In 1657 when Marmaduke Rawdon was injured in an accident (his coach overturned), his cousin, Mrs. Williams, cared for his injury with her "art" and he recovered in ten days.[62]

Dorothy Lawson, the wife of a barrister, ministered to the sick and needy in the area about her estate at Heaton in the county of Northumberland until her death in 1632.[63] Lady Honeywood, the wife of the local squire Sir Thomas Honeywood, was one of vicar Ralph Josselin's benefactresses who provided "divers things" for the treatment of Josselin's small daughter when she was very ill in 1645.[64] In 1648, Mrs. Josselin helped with the care of Honeywood's sick child, an example of how women exchanged medical assistance.[65] The same year, Lady Honeywood advised Josselin to treat his son with an "issue" whereby the bad humours could escape since she feared that he was "in a consumption."[66] When Josselin experienced pain and swelling after he removed the infected foot of a broken tooth, Lady Honeywood feared he had a "cancrish humour" and prescribed for him accordingly.[67] Mrs. Harlakenden was another gentlewoman who lived in Josselin's parish; she attempted to diagnose Mrs. Bettie's illness by viewing a sample of her urine which she also showed to Josselin, hoping to have him confirm her diagnosis.[68] Josselin credited his wife with successfully treating his children and himself on many occasions; his married daughter Jane continued the family tradition by providing her father with "syrup of pellitory" in 1677.[69]

The funeral eulogy of Lady Maynard in 1684 contained the following tribute:

She was a common patroness to the poor, and a common physician to her sick neighbours. Often she would with her own hands dress their most loathsome sores, and sometimes keep them in her home till cured.[70]

Hannah Woolley was another outstanding example of a successful female practitioner from late in the century. The author of a number of medical books, she dedicated one, published in 1680, "To all Ingenious Ladies and Gentlewoman."[71] Claiming that she had not only been a physician and surgeon to her own house, but also "to many of my Neighbours, eight or ten miles around," Woolley credited her early interest in 'physick and chirurgy' to her skilful mother and sisters. When Woolley was seventeen, she entered the employ of a "Noble Lady" who encouraged her interest by providing medical supplies as well as medicinal ingredients for the benefit of ailing neighbours. Her patroness bought medical books for Hannah, as well as obtaining direct information from physicians and surgeons of her acquaintance, for the young woman's benefit. After Woolley married the headmaster of a school, she continued to use her skills as a healer when students became ill, adding that the parents trusted her with all but desperately ill cases. Woolley believed that people should be able to treat themselves, but she stressed that difficult cures demanded good judgement as well as "Experience with much Reading."[72] Keeping in mind the limits imposed by available knowledge, her presentation, including case studies, was well-written and intelligently stated, making her a wonderful role model for women practitioners of her time. For example, Woolley noted that during her long experience as a physician and surgeon she had successfully cured cancer of the nose, cankers of the mouth and throat, green sickness, dropsy, jaundice, scurvy, vomiting, palsy and consumption. In a career which spanned some thirty-five years, she had also acquired surgical skills which enabled her to treat burns and scalds so that no scarring occurred.[73]

The account book of Sarah Fell contains numerous notations of expenditures for medicinal ingredients and treatments which the Fell sisters and their families used on their isolated estate in Cumberlandshire: oyl of almonds, innumerable quarts of white wine for "physick," turpentine, liquorice, vertigrass, a pound of allum for Richard Fell's leg, anniseeds, juniper and bayberries, treacle, tumeric, saffron and ale for a special drink known as Jannes drink (or Jane's Drink), purslane and cummin seeds.[74] Although the ingredients were most often for family members, the Fell family also looked after the needs of others such as Thomas Greaves' wife for whom they obtained one ounce of wormseed and "aloas," and Thomas Benson's ill wife for whom Sarah paid four pence for cinnamon.[75] Fennigreeke seeds to treat Pegg Gouth's knee cost two pence while Elizabeth Hopper reimbursed Sarah for the five shillings and five pence which she paid for a bottle of "burns water" for her.[76] In addition Sarah paid three pence for "bloodinge leeches" in 1674 on one occasion and 2 3/4 pence on another. In 1678, forty leeches cost four pence.[77] Sarah also mentioned purchasing "hiera picra," a preparation attributed to Galen which was made of aloes and myrrh.[78] From the entries in her account book, it is evident that Sarah and her sisters were adept at undertaking the role of both physician and surgeon.

On the other hand, although the women of the Ferrar family became proficient at treating surgical problems, they were forbidden to venture into physick by the family patriarch, Nicholas Ferrar.[79] The Ferrar women, who were literate and well-educated, made oils, salves and waters for "a great Surgions Chest" and under their mother's and uncle's instruction became very successful at treating even the most unpleasant sores and wounds. Even so, their uncle strictly forbade them to "meddle" with physick because it "required ye best art, long experience, deep judgement and no less Skill and mature Understanding." In other words, he perceived that his nieces lacked the qualities usually associated with the "superior" male psyche such as judgement and maturity, although they had demonstrated their technical skill in surgery. Even as his charges were encouraged to become proficient book-keepers "that they might have the knowledg and Skill of all that belonged to Housekeepers and good Housewifry," Nicholas restricted their practice of physick to the administration of nourishing broths to the sick poor, or "Kitchen Physick" as he called it.[80] The Ferrar family is a good example of how the range of women's knowledge and experience was circumscribed by the walls of their own households.[81] It also demonstrates why popular medicine, with its close association with the household or domestic milieu, was so widespread and why women were its foremost proponents.

The evidence for the role of female practitioners is limited by the nature of the sources. Undoubtedly a great deal of activity never came to be recorded in extant account books or correspondence; only a small minority kept diaries or made explicit reference to their own work or the efforts of their mothers or kinswomen. This stemmed, for the most part, from the fact that the practice was commonplace. For women lower down the social scale, the written evidence, by its very nature, is far more incomplete. Nevertheless, the indications all point to widespread involvement in popular medicine at this level. The nature of popular health care in seventeenth-century England can be usefully elaborated, however, through a study of educated, non-professional female use of herbals, receipt books and medical equipment, and through an analysis of the range and components of medical prescriptions and cures which can be traced to women.

Stuart gentlewomen generally owned equipment or "stills" which they used in the preparation of their various remedies. Descendants of the Verney family have given us the following description:

> The remains of queer tin vessels of many shapes with spouts at all angles in the ancient cupboards of the Claydon still-room, and the endless recipes among the papers, show how 'decoctions, infusions and essences of herbs and simples' were prepared.[82]

The Josselin family made use of home remedies on numerous occasions, a fact which stemmed in no small part from Mary Josselin's skill in distilling medicines. In 1646, Josselin mentioned the day in May on which she began to "still roses" and at various times, "syrup of roses," "rose ointment" and "oil of roses" were used to treat family illnesses.[83] Lady Margaret Hoby noted that she made "oile" in her closet and distilled waters such as aqua vita.[84] Lady Anne Clifford (Lady Hoby's cousin through marriage), described her mother's wide knowledge of "minerals, herbs, flowers and plants" and the "delight which she took in distilling waters and other chymical extractions."[85]

The role of the herbal in popular medicine was a crucial one since many of the medicines in everyday use involved the use of herbal ingredients. The use of herbals by women demonstrates the way popular practitioners relied upon both manuscript and published herbals for information about the herbs, plants, and roots which they used. One of the most famous of the herbals in use throughout the seventeenth century was John Gerard's *The Herball of General Historie of Plants*, more commonly known as Gerard's Herball, which was published in 1597.[86] In 1633 it appeared in an amended and enlarged form under the auspices of Thomas Johnson. John Parkinson was another botanical author of note who produced two valuable volumes in 1629 and 1640; John Symcotts, M.D., referred to both Gerard and Parkinson.[87] The most comprehensive bibliography of seventeenth-century herbals can be found in Eleanor Sinclair Rohde's *The Old English Herbals*. In it she lists manuscript herbals from the eleventh to the fifteenth centuries, as well as printed herbals. Of the latter, she shows twenty different titles for the seventeenth-century, exclusive of the numerous editions which some of the more popular herbals underwent, which underlines the continuing public demand for information of this nature throughout the seventeenth century.[88] In 1652 *Culpeper's Herbal* was published which was to prove so popular that over one hundred editions were eventually printed, most of them after 1700.[89] Evidently Ralph Josselin and his wife consulted both Gerard's and Culpeper's herbals. In 1650 he noted that his wife made him a syrup of "hissope" which eased his cough, while several decades later, they used burdock leaves to heal Ralph's sore legs.[90] Lady

Margaret Hoby consulted her herbal when she was actively engaged in treating the wounds and sores of servants and neighbours. She also gave away herbs from her own well-stocked herb garden and advised another female healer "a good wiffe of Erley [Everley]" on their use.[91] Much later in the century, Thomas Lawson, one of the most noted herbalists of his time, travelled to the isolated estate of the Fell family to instruct the sisters (as well as one of their husbands) on the use of herbs.[92]

On her journeys throughout England toward the end of the seventeenth century, Celia Fiennes showed a marked interest in stopping at herb gardens, among them the famous Physick Garden of Oxford.[93] Typical of the well-born women of her day, her knowledge of plants enabled her to comment at Windsor Castle on the "best maiden hairs, white and black, which is much esteemed for coughs and to put into drinks for consumption" and which was growing on the castle walls.[94] Fiennes also visited a well-to-do apothecary who showed her a "Herball" acquired from a Doctor of Physick.[95] This was not only an example of women's interest in herbs and herbals, it points out the way in which doctors and apothecaries, as well as women practitioners, relied on herbals for a good deal of their information.

Lady Mildmay was an elderly woman when she wrote in the seventeenth century about her early training during Elizabethan times at Lacock Abbey:

Also every day I spent some time in the Herball and books of Phisick and ministering to one or other by the directions of the best physicians of myne acquaintance; and ever God gave a blessing there unto.[96]

One twentieth-century researcher has commented on the "volumes of prescriptions, classified and carefully written in Lady Mildmay's own hand."[97] The same author, E.J. Cockram, concluded that information derived from country women was the source of many Elizabethan herbalists such as Brunfels, Cordus and Schneiburger.[98] Her conclusion is, however, unsubstantiated by documentation and therefore must remain in the realm of speculation.

The importance of medical books is also suggested by other individual cases relating to far from exceptional women. For example, the only possession specified in any detail in the 1654 will of Sarah Gater, the widow of a London merchant tailor, was her library, described in the following terms:

My Booke called Gerrards Herball withall my other Physick and Chirurgarie Books and notes and all my Bookes of Divinitie whatsoever not otherwise disposed of.[99]

Significantly, she bequeathed these all to her sister. At the other end of the social spectrum, the Verney family's "Aunt Isham," made out a list of bequests shortly before her death in 1667. In it, she left her "Herbal" to Lady Tipping who had earlier expressed a desire to have it, showing how highly valued these books were by women of wealth and standing.[100]

While country herb women or wise women depended for the most part on orally transmitted knowledge, many women of gentle birth could claim some degree of literacy and kept their own collections of "receipts" in personal "Receit Books." The practice of writing and preserving such books must have been widespread. For example, the Bedfordshire Record Office contains at least ten recipe books belonging to women; at least three are from the seventeenth century and four or five from the eighteenth century.[101] The persistence and continuity of this source of information for women practitioners is illustrated by the fact that the same office contains several books from the nineteenth century. Others are known to exist in various depositions. Several notable examples of female receipt books in manuscript can be found in the British Library, such as "Mary Doggett: Her Book of Receipts, 1682" and "My Lady Ranelagh's Choice Receipts" (undated), and in private collections. Of the latter, "The Lady Sedley's Receipt Book 1686" is a fine example.[102]

Although only a small number of these books have been printed, they are highly significant for advancing our knowledge of popular medicine and the role of women practitioners. Inasmuch as they contain cookery receipts as well as other information of a personal nature, their value in determining social attitudes towards health and medical conditions, for example female attitudes toward menstruation, is only beginning to be realized.[103] It should be pointed out that the practice of keeping receipt books was not limited exclusively to women. For instance a manuscript begun in 1589 at Anneville in Guernsey was compiled by succeeding generations of male members of the Andros family. Instead of the usual cookery receipts, it contained information on gardening, pruning and grafting interspersed with medical receipts.[104]

These receipt books were highly valued by their owners and contained prescriptions from a variety of sources: mothers, relatives, friends, servants, professional practitioners and authorities such as Gerard, author of the well-known herbal. One receipt book is known to have been passed down through six successive generations of females in a matriarchally linked family. The first known owner, Edith Beales, had been present in 1572 "att Paris in the massicar of St. Bartholumus day in the rain of Charles ye ninth of France." Additions had been made by other women in the family as it was passed from mother to daughter for almost 120 years.[105] Such a volume attests not only to the way medical knowledge was transmitted between women of each generation, but also to the great importance which members of society attached to these volumes.

Alice Thornton attempted to ensure that both of her daughters would carry on the traditions of home treatment already practised by both Alice and her mother. Her will, dated April 10, 1705, read in part:

Item I give unto my dear daughter Comber all my medicall books and Recepts, together with my stock of salves and oyntments, desireing her to give unto her sister Katherine Danby what she may have occasion to use for herself or her children.[106]

After Dame Margaret Verney's death in 1641, her will, drafted two years earlier, left the following instructions for her son Ralph:

...Now pray but non of my papers bee seene, but doe you burne them yrselfe. All but my noats and account and medsinable and coockery Boockes, such keep....[107]

Another example of the high esteem in which women's "receit" books were held can be found in the Barrington correspondence; in 1628, Sir Gilbert Gerard wrote his mother-in-law querying the whereabouts of some of his wife's books of "physicke." In particular, he wondered about "an old torne one [which] was left behind," and which must have been a favourite.[108]

An analysis of the receipts women used encompasses some 270 receipts culled from a variety of sources including women's personal receipt books, medical compendia containing receipts specifically attributed to women and contemporary letters and diaries. Three private receipt books contained a mixture of medicinal and cookery receipts; they yielded a total of 111 medicinal prescriptions.[109] The three medical compendia contained 150 prescriptions which were perceived as originating with female practitioners while the remaining dozen or so were found in other contemporary sources.[110] The receipts are of value for illustrating the wide range of illnesses which women treated. The largest number of receipts (38), were intended for what could be described as surgical conditions such as burns, wounds and atrophied sinews. For abnormalities of the gastro-intestinal tract (including the mouth), 28 receipts were offered while 27 were included for treating respiratory ailments including consumption. The great number of receipts for respiratory ailments and consumption is particularly significant in light of the fact that John Graunt's *Natural and Political Observations made upon the Bills of Mortality* lists these ailments as claiming the greatest number of lives of all causes in the thirty-year period 1629-1659.[111] Ophthalmic problems accounted for 16 prescriptions; for neurological problems such as headache, fainting and convulsions, 15 treatments were suggested. Only 13 of the receipts dealt with gynaecological problems including difficulties related to child birth. A possible explanation for this may have been the perception that midwives, whose knowledge was in an oral rather than written tradition, usually assumed responsibility for "female" ailments.[112] Other common ailments addressed in the receipts were: urological complaints, including the stone (12 receipts), circulatory and dropsy (9 receipts), plague, (13 receipts), sciatica and other aches and pains, (10 receipts), and gout, (5 receipts). At least one "cure" was included for food poisoning, hearing disorders, small pox, measles, ringworm, dermatological afflictions, corns, worms, King's Evil, jaundice, arthritis and chilblains. Thus it can be concluded that women practitioners were actively engaged in treating a broad spectrum of medical and surgical problems, including those with the highest mortality rates.

In addition to the women's receipts which were designated to treat specific medical conditions, there are prescriptions for salves, ointments, purges, diet drinks, "opening mixtures," cordials, emulsions, oils, waters and glysters, to be used at the healer's discretion. Each receipt book contains at least one "polychrest" or universal medicine which could be used for a whole host of conditions. For example, Lady Jane's "walnutt" water (which could be taken internally or applied externally), could be given for fevers, poor appetite, palsy, dropsy, sore eyes, insomnia, whitening the skin, abscesses, wounds (including infected flesh), obstructions in the stomach caused by overindulgence in food and drink, small pox, and the promotion of longevity. Many of the receipts came with specific, often quite complex, directions for the preparation of the ingredients. Lady Jane's walnut water gave alternative instructions for green or ripe walnuts; of the latter she wrote:

take 300 wallnutts on St. John's day, bruis them in a mortar and lay them in 2 qts best white wine vinegar, let them ly 3 days & then distill them at St. James' tide. Take 300 more, bruis them & still them when they are full ripe. Take as many more, bruis them, hull & shells and together & still them all together the 3d. water.[113]

Even more complex was Lady Hewet's cordial water which contained seventy-two ingredients. It was offered with the following comment:

This is an excellent cordiall, good for a great many distempers, it will presarve life a few minuets longer, in any dieing pesson if you give them some of it - it will cost 50 shillings a quart to make it.[114]

Receipts such as this illustrate the time, effort and expense involved in preparing many of the prescriptions. They also underline the dedication, not to mention the skill, with which Stuart gentlewomen undertook the task of ministering to the health needs of their contemporaries.

Several conclusions can be drawn from an examination of women's receipts. The predominant impression is that women's receipts were virtually no different from those used by male practitioners (professional and lay) both in the complexity of their ingredients and the imprecision with which they were assigned to various disease and ailments. For example the prescription for "Dr. Stephen's water" appeared in Susanna Avery's book, Diana Astry's book and Lady Sedley's receipt book. Lady Sedley described it as a 'polychrest' remedy, good for treating a variety of conditions including halitosis and barrenness.[115]

In the light of twentieth-century knowledge, only a very few women's receipts could have had a beneficial effect; Alice Thornton's treatment of her mother's pneumonia with poultices to her chest was a useful measure.[116] Lady Mildmay's "drink for a Cough or Cold," contained liquorice, aniseeds and honey, all ingredients of modern cough remedies.[117] Lady Nevill's treatment for inflammation of the breast using a poultice of beans and linseed was an effective treatment.[118] These, however, were the exception rather than the rule. In addition, the evidence is of necessity biased toward upper-class women. Perhaps the treatments used by country women were simpler, perhaps they were more generally efficacious; but since there are few written records of them, such speculation must remain unsupported. Although reformers such as Noah Biggs eulogized the past and claimed for it a simpler, more natural knowledge (including medical knowledge), the few folk remedies and receipts which we have such as three or four from the Dorset region, as well as several which bear designations usually associated with women of humble origins, do not differ significantly from many other women's receipts.

Despite the limitations inherent in women's exclusion from "formal" medical studies, women authors made a significant contribution to the corpus of medical literature associated with the seventeenth century. In addition to a large number of receipt books in manuscript authored by females, a posthumous collection of receipts attributed to the Countess of Kent was first published in 1653. It subsequently underwent 19 editions in the next 34 years. One of its seventy odd receipts was for the popular Countess of Kent's Powder which was notable for the inclusion of crab's eyes and claws among its ingredients. A polychrest medication, it could be used to treat French pox, small pox, measles, plague, scarlet fever, malignant fever and melancholic.[119]

Female practitioner Hannah Woolley was also an author of note. Her book *The Accomplish'd Lady's Delight in preserving, beautifying, cookery and gardening* underwent nine printings between 1670 and 1706.[120] One of her books, *The Queen-like Closet* (1674) was translated into German and published in Hamburg in 1697. She authored at least four other books (including one on angling), all of which received wide acceptance.[121] Mary Trye was also a female practitioner. She was the author of *Mediatrix or the Woman Physician* and carried on the work of her father, deceased chemical physician Thomas O'Dowd. Trye continued to champion her father's cause eight years after his death and levelled charges at Dr. Henry Stubbs, a Warwick physician, for his use of phlebotomy to treat scurvy and small pox. Trye challenged Stubbs to a trial of their respective cures, offering to cure two patients (without using the lancet) to every one which Stubbs attempted to cure using the Galenic regimen.[122]

After a promising start which urged women "not to let their great worth with other learned authors of our sex ly in obscurity," Sarah Ginnor, self-styled "Student of Physick," wrote what became little more than a parody of astrological physicians.[123] She did, however, acknowledge the "great and wonderful" cures done by her sex and generally supported the view that women were not only competent, but knowledgeable practitioners.

In view of the activity of women medical authors of manuscript, as well as printed, receipt books, assertions that the increasing literacy of housewives and gentlewomen undermined traditional medicine and led to the decline of traditional (popular) practitioners, are questionable.[124] This conclusion was reached by Harold Cook but the opposite conclusion is indicated by the evidence; literacy helped to preserve and disseminate medical information from earlier generations of lay practitioners, especially female practitioners.

Comments by informed contemporaries leave no doubt as to the extensive role played by non-professional women in health care. The appropriateness of their role was, however, an issue for debate. A study of the controversy sheds considerable light upon the attitudes towards, as well as the prevalence of, popular medicine in this period. Hostility towards uneducated female practitioners was limited to the medical profession itself. Even here, there was a mixed response. A number of physicians (including some of the most militant medical reformists), accepted the traditional role of females in the provision of health care or argued for the expansion of their activity by advocating the supplementation of their medical knowledge. Complaints were, for the most part, limited to specific cases. Throughout the century, informally educated gentlewomen and illiterate wise women co-existed with the professional elite in serving the health needs of the population.[125]

One of the strongest attacks on female practitioners came from physician John Cotta whose book on "Ignorant Practisers of Physicke," published in 1612, devoted a chapter to women. Cotta began by pointing out women's lack of formal education, a handicap, which he argued, could almost never be overcome despite hard work and any natural abilities a women might possess. In addition, Cotta questioned women's capacity for "learned reason and understanding" in matters of life and death; such deficiencies were inherent afflictions, according to Cotta, bestowed by "God and Nature."[126] Cotta denounced the dangerous practices of women practitioners, such as the daily administration of laxatives to an elderly man for a period of ten days.[127] He also criticized women who offered advice on medical matters, citing those who dissuaded a gentlewomen from having a phlebotomy; Cotta felt such a measure would have saved her life.[128] Cotta denigrated the domestic nature of women's practice and went so far as to assert that everyday household dietary items such as milk, butter, broth, meat and juices could be dangerous if used inappropriately.[129] Despite the harsh rhetoric which Cotta directed toward female practitioners, his criticism in some instances became an eloquent, if unintentional, testimonial to their empirically-based abilities and treatments:

...because by time and custome they are become familiarly knowne unto them, and now are of their owne domesticall preparations, & therefore are by their knowledge, acquaintance, and avouching of them, growne into some credite and reputation with them.[130]

Although Cotta obscured his real concern by trying to show that uneducated women practioners were dangerous, it was not the public as much as the pocketbooks of the professionals he wished to protect.[131] For instance, the few isolated examples of female malpractice which he cited were, for the most part, less serious than instances of malpractice by male professionals which have come to our attention.[132]

There were other members of the medical profession who obviously perceived the threat which women posed to their own status and income. One treatise which was addressed to women undoubtedly had the interests of the professionals in mind. *The Sicke Womans Private Looking Glass* (1636) featured the picture of a woman consulting a male doctor and on the opposite page, a poem:

The Strength of Herbs and
planets influence
Physicians skill, through Gods
benevolence
To young and old, to husband and to wife
Are the appointed meanes for a healthfull life.[133]

Having limited the practice of medicine to physicians with a knowledge of herbs and astrology, John Sadler, a physician from Norwich, went on to point out that women's "ignorance and modesty" deterred them from consulting physicians. His aim, he claimed, was to inform women about signs and symptoms of female diseases so that they could consult a (male) physician and receive treatment when it was warranted. Sadler warned against self-treatment which could aggravate the disease. More than twenty years later, John Tanner adopted somewhat different tactics in an attempt to curtail women's practice. He wrote that his aim was: "To help Ladies and gentlewomen who are wont to help their poor sick neighbours" to recognize dangerous symptoms which require a physician's intervention, and "that all women may the better understand the Physitians Directions and with more Prudence govern the sick."[134] Tanner hoped to ensure that women's role as practitioners would become merely an adjunct to that of the doctor. This would result in an undermining of women's confidence in their traditional role of healer and increase their dependence on a male medical profession who claimed an expertise based on "formal" medical education.

Physician Richard Whitlock published *Zootomia* in 1654. It is a collection of medical satires which, while unofficial, can be taken as representative of the views of the College of Physicians, according to Christopher Bentley.[135] Whitlock's attack on "shee-physitians" is particularly vitriolic, accusing them of killing, rather than curing, their patients. His description of non-professionals, including women, follows:

All that falsely usurp this title of Physitian, and practice it, to the sad cost of many;... Wicked Jewes, Murtherers of Christians, Monks, abdicant of their orders, &c. Unlearned Chymists, conceited Pedagogues, dull Mechanicks, Pragmaticall Barbers, wandring Mountebancks, Cashiered Souldiers, indebted Trades-men, Husband-men.... Toothlesse women, fudling Gossips, and Chare-women, talkative midwives, &c. In summe...the scum of Mankind.[136]

Richard Banister, surgeon and oculist, shared the view of Cotta and others that women's lack of formal education led to malpractice. Despite his apparent hostility to women practitioners as a whole, Banister accepted gentlewomen practitioners who treated the poor, "not for gain." Further inconsistencies in his view of women are revealed by Banister's account of an unnamed woman at Joynville who was able to remove parasites from a man's eye with a silver needle after a surgeon had failed to help the man. Banister added "The woman said she had done this previously for many others with no hurt ensuing." Also cited favourably by Banister was a woman "famous for curing the Scorby."[137] Banister then was clearly inconsistent, insisting on one hand upon the need for theoretical knowledge, but on the other hand accepting the value of popular practitioners in individual cases.

Most of the "average" physicians like John Symcotts, M.D., accepted the role of women practitioners, even to the extent of adopting their treatments. As noted above, when in 1636 one of his patients was suffering from puerpera as a complication of pregnancy, he used a broth made of shepherd's purse which had been suggested by a beggar woman; he subsequently used the same "cure" for other patients.[138] Symcotts also used receipts which were given to him by gentlewomen as well as noting cures by women; for example, the two treatments used by Mrs. Corbet and Mistress Child, respectively, for the cure of umbilical hernias in children.[139] Physician Martin Blockwich wrote approvingly of a country woman who was skilled in treating cases of ascites and stone.[140]

Medical literature from the period indicates an acceptance of women's role as non-professional medical practitioners and in some cases approval and encouragement from the professionals themselves.[141] In 1651, Leonard Sowerby published *The Ladies Dispensatory containing the Natures, Vertues and Qualities of All herbs and Simples usefull in Physick.* In the foreward he stressed the fact that it contained straightforward, elementary medicines which were unsophisticated and easily grasped since they were all in the English language.[142] A 1651 edition of Vicary's *The Surgions Directorie* was published by T.F. who added as a subtitle: "As a noble Exercise for Gentlewomen, and others; who desire Science in Medicine and Surgery, for a generall Good." He reiterated his intention in the foreward: "To all vertuous Ladyes & Gentlewomen of this Commonwealth of England" and closed by saying "Thus leaving you Ladies and Gentlewomen to your chairitable acting and doing good when need shall require."[143]

The year 1657 saw the publication of *De Morbis Foemines The Womans Counsellor: or the Feminine Physitian,* intended for medical students, maids, wives, widows and midwives. Written as a self-help book because of women's "excess modesty," it must have disappointed many women who purchased it in order to acquire practical information on gynaecological disorders. In addition to an assortment of remedies which would have been of no help to female sufferers, the author suggested that "If the Patient be a Maid, a Husband is the best medicine."[144] *The Child bearers Cabinet* was the first sub-title of *A Rich Closet of Physical Secrets,* published in 1652, making it clearly a publication directed to a female audience.[145] The author of *Nature Exenterata* published in 1655, dedicated his book to "Gentlemen, Ladies and others." This book (discussed earlier in the chapter), contained contributions by 44 women, who were identified in the "Index." They included the Countess of Surrey, whose picture graced the frontispiece.[146] When Robert Pemell published the second edition of *Tractus De facultatibus Simplicium* in 1653, he included a tract entitled *De Morbis Puerorum; or a Treatise of the Diseases of Children With their Causes, Signs, Prognosticks and Cures, for the benefit of such as do not understand the Latine Tongue, and very usefull for all such as are House-Keepers and have Children.*[147] Edward Poeton dedicated *The Chyrurgeons Closet* to Francis, Countess of Exeter, in 1630 with a flowery tribute which read in part:

where is there any woman living, that hath spent so much time in the study of this art and made so gracious & painful a progress in the practice thereof, as your thrice noble selfe. Do not the soules of the sick and sore & the limbs of the lame, everywhere (where ere you reside) bless you.[148]

Thomas Collins dedicated his book on Physicke and Surgery to "the honourable and truly vertuous gentlewoman, Mistress Ursula Bucke."[149] Dedications such as these indicate that medical treatises were deemed highly appropriate for the literate gentlewomen. Although not specifically addressed to women, *The Doctresse*, (by Bunworth), *A Collection of Rare and Select Secrets in Physick and Chyrurgery, Collected and Practised by the Right Honourable, the Countesse of Kent, late deceased*, as well as *The Queen's Closet opened* would all attract a female readership by their titles which were of obvious interest to women.[150] Further evidence that women's interest in medical treatises was not limited to those specifically intended for their use can be found in female ownership inscriptions. For example, George Thomson's *Galeno-Pale* is inscribed with the name "Jane Papillon."[151]

While the general response of the typical physician was one of acceptance with regard to female non-licensed practitioners (especially those of the upper class), a small group of medical reformers adopted a more positive attitude toward women healers. While it must be borne in mind that in the case of two of the reformers, Noah Biggs and George Starkey, their aim was to point out the deficiencies of traditional Galenic medicine and the strengths of the Paracelsian school, their assessment of female practitioners was laudatory. Noah Biggs wrote of "old women" bold enough to venture into "the practice of Physick"..."putting an affront upon Physitians because of times in many things they excele them."[152] Starkey argued that a doctor's cure for gout was no better than one by a "good old woman;" he also believed that women's cures were greatly undervalued, pointing out that while a woman who used simple, natural cures could hardly expect thanks, the same cure by a doctor would be regarded as a miracle.[153] The most outstanding medical reformer, critic and author of the period was Nicholas Culpeper. In his famous translation of the *London Dispensatory*, he made it clear that his intended audience included "Gentlewomen who freely bestow your pains, brains and cost to your poor wounded and diseased neighbours."[154] Culpeper also published *A Directory for Midwives* in 1651. This was reprinted no less than 17 times, the last time in 1777.[155] Indeed Culpeper's whole aim was:

not to make fools physicians, but to help those that are ingenious, rational and industrious though they have not the knowledge of tongues that were to be desired.[156]

Although Culpeper intended to serve the interests of the public at large by his translations, women who were traditionally denied the benefit of formal education in the classical tongues were his greatest beneficiaries.

Throughout the seventeenth century, educated non-professionals readily accepted the role of female non-professionals. In 1651, Gervase Markham published his book *Country Contentments* which contained a section entitled "The English Housewife." He outlined what was expected of every gentlewoman with regard to preventive medicine as well as medical treatment; his commentary not only captured the climate of the time, it also reflected many of the actual household practices outlined above:

> To beginne with then with one of the most principall vertues which doth belong to our English hous-wife; you shall understand that the preservation and care of the familie touching their health and soundesse of bodie consisteth most in her diligence: it is meet that shee have a phisicall kinde of knowledge, how to administer many wholsome receipts or medicines for the good of their healthes, as well to prevent the first occasion of sicknesse, as to take away the effects and evill of the same when it hath made seizure on the body.[157]

The expectation that gentlewomen would have some knowledge of home remedies prevailed throughout the century moving Richard Allestree, who published *The Ladies Calling* in 1673, to laud the compassion of wealthy women who had formerly attended the sick and needy at their own expense and to urge all well-born women to emulate their example:

> ...not only opening up their purses, but dispensatories too, providing medicines for such as either by disease or casualty want that sort of relief... & instead of repairing or disguising their own complexions, study the restauration of their decrepit patients limbs.[158]

Robert Boyle, eminent scientist and philosopher, wrote of "ladies and old wives" who performed "more constant and easy cures than learned physicians."[159] One of the leading intellectuals of the century, Thomas Hobbes, had little faith in medication. When he was forced, on occasion, to seek medical advice, "he preferred an 'experienced old woman' to the most learned and inexperienced physician."[160]

Although the Verney family could boast an M.D. as one of its members, it frequently used prescriptions or remedies supplied by "ordinary" women. In 1647, Sir Ralph Verney, wrote to his wife with a request for two prescriptions.

> There is an excellent medicine that Mrs. Francis was wont to make for the cankar 'twas black and boyled in an egg shell... also the receipt of goodwife Greene's medicine for a pinn and webb in the eye... 'tis made of soures and severall herbes, and is

to bee drunke. parhapps Dr. will laugh at it but I know tis good, and have found it soe myself.[161]

It is highly significant that Sir Ralph, himself a university graduate who had recourse to the services of an excellent physician by contemporary standards, had more confidence in the "cures" of a popular practitioner than in the good doctor's. In 1664, Sir Ralph's son Edmund was at his wits' end because of his wife's persistently recurring mental illness. A woman named Clark was recommended to him who would undertake a two-month treatment for a fee of £20; reputedly the woman had successfully treated a thirteen-year-old girl with a similar complaint. When Edmund sought his father's advice in the matter, Sir Ralph commented "divers Woemen have very good receipts and good successe too & frequently have cured those that the Drs. have not."[162] Evidently Edmund decided to employ 'the woman Dr.' and his wife Mary experienced temporary improvement. By 1671, Edmund was again seeking help for his wife; he consulted Widow Scott or 'old Judith' who attempted a cure by binding the head of a jack hare "wrapt in something" to her patient's head for several days and nights.[163] When Ralph Verney suffered a troublesome eruption on his leg and thigh, his friends recommended an ointment concocted by "a dreadful old woman."[164] Sir Ralph wrote to his wife in 1647 about their ailing three-week-old child, demonstrating again that he valued the expertise of women healers:

give the child no physick but such as midwives and old women, with the doctor's approbation, doe prescribe; for assure yourself they by experience know better than any phisition how to treat such infants.[165]

Earlier in the century, the family of Simon D'Ewes shared similar confidence in female practitioners' skill with infants and left its young son Simon in the care of Mrs. Margaret Waltham of Dorchester after he ruptured himself by crying.[166]

Alice Thornton of Yorkshire, whose husband was a member of the minor gentry, consulted Dr. Wittie for family illnesses on occasion. However in 1667 when her daughter Nally had a "pearle on her eye" as the result of smallpox, she called on "sweate Mis Bucke" who saved the child's eyesight, according to Alice, by the use of "waters and a medicine," the latter applied to the wrists.[167] Elias Ashmole also consulted physicians for various problems but in 1647 when his toes were infected, he used oil and salve from a Mrs. Stafford to effect a cure.[168] When Ralph Josselin's wife was ill, he sent for a neighbour woman such as Mrs. Mabel, who came and ministered unto her.[169] Adam Martindale described his amazing cure by a "poore woman" who used a salve made of celadine, the moss of an ash root, and May butter after "skillful men, or so esteemed" had failed to cure a "vehement fermentation" and widespread "ugly dry scurfe."[170] Gentlewoman Lucy Hutchinson, herself a healer of note, disclosed the fact that her maid went to another town to have her sore eye cured by a townswoman there, a significant testimony to the skill of the unnamed woman.[171] The Pelhams and the Dacres of Sussex, both "major gentry households," used the services of local herb women to supplement "official" medical practitioners, in cases of family illness.[172] The actions of a wide variety of well-educated and intelligent individuals of this period, therefore, demonstrate a ready acceptance of the significant role played by unofficial, possibly illiterate, female healers within this society.

In conclusion, women's role in Stuart medicine was not limited to either the few country wise women nor the occasional gentlewomen who have surfaced in the traditional studies of the seventeenth century. Examination of a variety of sources throughout the century supports the view that women of all social ranks were actively engaged in carrying out surgical and medical treatment for a broad spectrum of ailments throughout urban and rural England. Women's practice (which in many cases used the same treatments as the professionals) was generally of a high quality, given the limits of contemporary medical knowledge. This fact was recognized by the general public as well as the medical profession, with a few exceptions. Taken in a wider context, the case of Stuart women as practitioners of popular medicine illustrates the widespread nature of popular medicine, its quality, diversity, acceptance and the valuable role it filled in the delivery of health care throughout the seventeenth century.

Conclusion

Aside from one or two local studies, historians of early modern medicine have generally accepted a model of English health care which concentrated on professional practitioners and practice. They have at the same time admitted the presence of an undefined group of simple, country healers who were located mainly in the provinces. According to this prevailing concept, the professionals acted as the leaders in medical inquiry and expertise as well as the sustainers of the burden of health care. To the extent that non-professionals have attracted the attention of scholars, the historical literature has been mixed. Many historians have simply adopted the contemporary views of the College of Physicians and several notable publicists which equated unlicensed practitioners with quacks; others have perceived the country "wise" people as drawing upon an exclusively "natural" knowledge based on an extensive familiarity with common herbs and plants. This simple, pure folklore was seen as a noble, if inferior, substitute for the services of the educated, licensed professional.

An examination of a variety of sources, however, has led to the conclusion that twentieth-century perceptions have strongly influenced medical historians and created a largely simplistic, dichotomized view of medical practice. The assumption that there existed a body of superior, scientific medical knowledge accessible only to educated, trained professionals is untenable, as is a conception of popular medicine as being in essence illiterate folk remedies. Scholars have, perhaps unconsciously, viewed popular lay care as "fringe" or "alternative" medicine because of the biases inherent in a modern perspective. In quantitative terms, popular practice was at the centre of health care, not its fringe; in qualitative terms, there was surprisingly little difference in most respects between the content and practice of these two sectors of health care.

Several factors contributed to the marginalization of popular medicine and the unsubstantiated belief that it was either inconsequential or in rapid decline in the seventeenth century. One is the methodological problem engendered by the historiographical emphasis upon charting the increasing knowledge, sophistication and organization of the medical profession, and in particular the elite graduate physicians. Another is the assumption that increasing literacy spelt the end of folk medicine.

This study demonstrates that both beliefs are founded upon a faulty understanding of popular medicine and its place within seventeenth-century health care. Chapter one has rejected the arguments of R.S. Roberts that supply and demand worked against popular practitioners and increasingly displaced them from practice in early Stuart England. Here, and in Chapter two, it has been demonstrated how professional practice was, in the main, limited to a small percentage of the prosperous, and, to some extent, urban population. Even within this elite sector of society, self-treatment and reliance upon traditional practitioners were commonplace. Chapter three added the powerful incentive of religion for the retention of traditional medicine, and demonstrated the extent of the intellectual contrivances of physicians, hardpressed to justify their very existence. Chapter four documented the absence of a body of "scientific" knowledge which was the exclusive preserve of the professional. Nor was there a body of "pure" lay knowledge. The treatments and medications used by many lay and professional practitioners were virtually the same, each group adding to and borrowing from the "receipts" of the other. For this reason (as well as the limitations imposed by contemporary medical knowledge), neither lay nor professional could demonstrate a clear superiority in treating illness. Women of all social classes have emerged as leading proponents of popular medicine and as a major segment of its practitioners. A case study of their role, in Chapter five, demonstrated the widespread and diverse nature of popular medicine as it was practised throughout society.

Historians have been too ready to adopt a "Whiggish" perspective of seventeenth-century medicine. The period of the notable medical discoveries of Harvey, Glisson and Ent, Sydenham and Willis cannot be viewed as the direct precursor of the twentieth century, without some distortion of the evidence and the dismissal of an entire sector of traditional health care. However valuable these scientific discoveries were, it has not yet been demonstrated that they revolutionized medicine at the clinical level during the seventeenth century.[1] Further, there is no proof that this research was even necessarily representative of the majority view within the medical profession itself. The very slow and unenthusiastic acceptance, even in principle, of Harvey's theory of the circulation of the blood, for example, is well known.[2] To interpret Stuart medicine solely from the perspective of a medical profession which was assumed to be in control of a superior body of knowledge and expertise is therefore unacceptable.

A revised and realistic appraisal of the role of popular medicine which places it at the centre of seventeenth-century health care suggests other topics within the broad framework of popular medicine which would contribute to our knowledge and understanding of medical practice and health care as a whole. Out of our current research the female practitioner stands in need of further investigation. Matriarchally disseminated medical knowledge as well as the role of literacy in the practice of popular medicine both merit further investigation. A new perspective for seventeenth-century medicine opens the way to fresh avenues of research. In particular, by shifting the focus of the history of medicine away from a small body of professionals, attention is drawn to the need to establish health care within its social context, as a vital and integral aspect of the social and intellectual world of early modern English men and women. The study of non-professional practitioners and the non-professional aspect of medicine has the potential to reveal far more about this society than does the hitherto exclusive inquiry into the rise of a profession.

As an example of the broader utility inherent within a re-orientated conception of Stuart medicine, one could refer to the topic of radicalism and intellectual ferment during the revolutionary era, 1641-60. Christopher Hill, in particular, has interpreted the strength of popular medicine in this period as a reaction against established professionalism, and as an integral part of radical demands for the end of intellectual monopolies in medicine, the church and the legal profession.[3] According to Hill's paradigm, popular medicine was novel, radical and antithetical toward established authorities and norms. Yet, although a few "radicals" made their views heard during this period, a longer time frame demonstrates no evidence of significant change in either the character or incidence of popular medicine.[4] Professor Hill's interpretation is founded upon a misunderstanding of the nature of popular medicine and is premised upon the belief that the professionals already possessed a monopoly of medicine in the early Stuart era. Since this was not the case, the facile relationship drawn with the clergy and legal profession is unproductive. Evidence throughout the century points to continuity in practice and ideas.[5]

In conclusion, then, this detailed study of seventeenth-century popular medicine supports the view that a widespread system of health care existed alongside the small corps of a medical elite, traditionally credited with providing health care in England. The quality and character of health care provided by popular practitioners was virtually indistinguishable from that given by the professionals. This "unofficial" system of health care was administered by a large number of lay practitioners and was central to, rather than an adjunct of, "professional" medical practice.

Notes

Notes to Introduction

[1]Nancy G. Siraisi, "Some Current Trends in the Study of Renaissance Medicine," *Renaissance Quarterly* 37 (Winter 1984): 585-600.

[2]Ibid., pp. 590-91. See Margaret Pelling "Occupational Diversity: Barber Surgeons and the Trades of Norwich, 1550-1640," *Bulletin of the History of Medicine* 56 (1982): 484-511.

[3]Ibid., 599. While Siraisi is right to encourage the examination of physicians' records and correspondence, by narrowing her perspective to intellectual history she misses the value of these documents for social historians. For examples of how these can be used, see below, the casebooks of Symcotts and Hall.

[4]Roy Porter, "Was there a Medical Enlightenment in Eighteenth-century England?" *British Journal for Eighteenth-Century Studies* 5 (1982): 49-63 and Porter, "Lay Medical Knowledge in the Eighteenth-century: The Evidence of the Gentlemen's Magazine" *Medical History* 29 (1985): 133-168.

[5]R.S. Roberts, "The Personnel and Practice of Medicine in Tudor and Stuart England," *Medical History* 6 (1962): 363-382; 8 (1964): 217-234. See also T.D. Whittet, "The apothecary in Provincial Gilds," *Medical History* 8 (1964): 245-273; Sidney Young, *The Annals of the Barber Surgeons of London* (London: Blades, East and Blades 1890).

[6]John H. Raach, *A Directory of English Country Physicians 1603-1643* (London: Dawson's of Pall Mall, 1962).

[7]Charles Webster, *The Great Instauration: Science, Medicine and Reform 1626-1660* (London: Duckworth, 1975).

[8]Siraisi, p. 97. For other examples of this genre, see Kenneth Dewhurst, "Thomas Sydenham (1624-1689) Reformer Of Clinical Medicine" *Medical History* 6 (1962): 101-118; B.A. Shaw, "Sir Thomas Browne," *British Medical Journal* 285, 1 (1982): 40-42.

[9]See for example Phyllis Allen, "Medical education in 17th Century England," *Journal of the History of Medicine and Allied Sciences* 1 (January 1946): 115-143; James L. Axtell, "Education and Status in Stuart England: The London Physician," *History of Education Quarterly* 10, (1970): 141-59. Axtell presents an extremely romanticized, Whiggish view of the attainments of the seventeenth-century medical profession; A.H.T. Robb-Smith "Medical Education at Oxford and Cambridge Prior to 1850." in F.N.L. Poynter (ed.), *The Evolution of Medical Education in Britain* (London: Pitman Medical Publishing Co. Ltd., 1966); J.J. Keevill, "The Seventeenth century English Medical Background," *Bulletin of the History of Medicine* 31 (1957): 408-424. See also Harold John Cook, "The Regulation of Medical Practice in London under the Stuarts 1607-1704." (Ph.D. Dissertation, University of Michigan, 1981) for how the College acted to promote and protect the interests of this small group of physicians.

[10]Robert Frank, "The Physician as Virtuoso in Seventeenth-Century England," in B. Shapiro and R. Frank (eds.) *English Virtuosi in the Sixteenth and Seventeenth Centuries* (Los Angeles: University of California Press, 1979), p. 178-179.

[11]For an example of the historian who saw this positive course for seventeenth century medicine see Lester S. King, *The Road to Medical Enlightenment 1650-1695* (London: MacDonald, 1970).

[12]Margaret Pelling, Charles Webster "Medical Practitioners" in Webster (ed.), *Health, Medicine and Mortality in the Sixteenth Century* (Cambridge: Cambridge University Press, 1979, pp. 165-235), p. 235.

[13]Roy Porter, "One man's herb, another man's medicine," *The Listener* (June 23, 1983): 14-16 (p. 14). Porter suggests all of these alternative designations for popular medicine. See also W.F. Bynum, Roy Porter (eds.), *Medical Fringe and Medical Orthodoxy 1750-1850.* (Beckenham, Kent: Croom Helm, 1987) for evidence of the enduring nature of unlicensed practice.

[14]Sir George Clark, *A History of the Royal College of Physicians of London* 2 Vols. (Oxford: Clarendon Press, 1964).

[15]Christopher Hill, *Change and Continuity in Seventeenth-Century England* (London: Weidenfeld and Nicolson, 1974, pp. 157-178).

[16]Matthew Ramsey, "Medical Power and Popular Medicine," *Journal of Social History* 10 (1976): 560-587.

[17]Pelling and Webster, "Medical Practitioners", p. 166.

[18]Porter, "One man's herb", p. 14. For other views on quacks and quackery, see Herbert Silvette, "On Quacks and Quackery in Seventeenth-Century England," *Annals of Medical History*, 3rd Series, 1 (1939): 239-251; William B. Ober, "Noble Quacksalver: The Earl of Rochester's Merry Prank," *History of Medicine* 2 (1973): 24-26. Hector A. Colwell, "Lionel Lockyer," *Proceedings of the Royal Society of Medicine* 3 (1915): 126-34; James Bishop, "John Archer's Secrets Disclosed'," *Tubercle* (London) 38 (1957): 432-5. Leslie G. Matthews, "Licensed Mountebanks in Britain," *Journal of the History of Medicine* 19 (1964): 30-45. Gordon W. Jones, "A Relic of the Golden Age of Quackery: What Read Wrote," *Bulletin of the History of Medicine* 37 (1963): 226-238. For examples of advertisements by quacks, see Salvator Winter Maretto, *Advertisement* (London, 1647; Thomason E 526 (19)) and Peter Francesse, *Advertisement,* (London, 1656; Thomason E 93).

[19]For a description of the episcopal licensing system, including verbatim transcript, see John R. Guy, "The Episcopal Licensing of Physicians, Surgeons and Midwives," *Bulletin of the History of Medicine* 56 (1982): 528-542.

Chapter 1

[1]R.S. Roberts, "Medicine in Tudor and Stuart England. Part I The Provinces," *Medical History* 6, (1962), p. 369.

[2]John H. Raach, *A Directory*, p. 14 and Peter Heath, *The Parish Clergy on the Eve of the Reformation* (London, Routledge and Kegan Paul, 1969), p. 24.

[3]Raach, *A Directory*. Since most of the physicians in Raach's study practiced for only a fraction of the forty years, the number of parishes per physician would be far greater.

[4]Margaret Pelling and Charles Webster, "Medical Practitioners," p. 188.

[5]Christopher Hill, *Change and Continuity*, p. 157. Robb-Smith, "Medical Education at Oxford and Cambridge." p. 49.

[6]Lady Margaret Hoby, Dorothy Meads, ed., *Diary of Lady Hoby* (Boston & N.Y.: Houghton Mifflin Co., 1930), pp. 149, 202, 214. According to the *OED*, physick was a cathartic or purge. In keeping with the humoral theory upon which the medical practice of the day was founded, Lady Hoby and her husband would submit to purging in an attempt to rid themselves of possible accumulations of bad "humours". It is an interesting commentary on medicine as it was practiced, that in each instance, Lady Hoby's diary recorded the fact that she was always much sicker after her treatment than she was before it.

[7]Simon Haward, *Phlebotomy: Or, A Treatise of Letting Blood* (London: 1601; S.T.C. 12922; Reprinted., N.Y.: Da Capo Press, 1973).

[8]*Calendar of State Papers, Domestic Series, reign of Charles I, vol. 18 (1640), p.280.*

[9]Arthur Searle, ed. *Barrington Family Letters 1628-1632* (Camden Society, 4th series, vol. 28: London: The Royal Historical Society, 1983), p. 144.

[10]Raach, *A Directory*, p. 110.

[11]See Margaret Pelling, "Occupational Diversity: Barber Surgeons and the Trades of Norwich, 1550-1640," *Bulletin of the History of Medicine* 56 (1982): 484-511.

[12]Medical literature throughout the seventeenth century stressed the importance of supervision by a physician while "taking the waters", internally or externally. See Tobias Venner, *Via recta ad vitam longam* (London, 1650; Thomason Tracts E6051). This was originally printed in 1620 with an appended section on "the bathes of Bathe"; Eugenius Philander, *Drinking of Bath Waters* (London, 1673; Wing P 1984), pp. 14-22; Thomas Guidat, *The Register of Bath* (London, 1694; Wing G 2199), which deals with scores of reputed cures for a variety of illnesses over a 27 year period, and Robert Pierce, *Bath Memoirs* (Bristol, 1697), "The Preface." See also John French, M.D., *The Yorkshire Spaw* (London, 1652; Thomason F 2175) and Celia Fiennes, ed., Christopher Morris, *The Journeys of Celia Fiennes* (London: Cresset Press, 1949), pp. 17-21, for a full account of a lay person's perception of the ritual involved in "taking the bathes".

[13]Raach, *A Directory*, p. 113 and R.S. Neale, *Bath 1680-1850: A Social History* (1981), p. 44 in David Underdown, *Revel, Riot and Rebellion: Popular Politics and Culture in England, 1603-1660* (Oxford: Clarendon, 1985) p. 294n. Even taking into account the seasonal influx of visitors to the waters, the high ratio of doctor to patient is obvious, especially since some visitors were accompanied by their own physicians; see note 15 below.

[14]R.Pierce, *Bath Memoirs* "The Preface" and p. 389.

[15]Harriet Joseph, *Shakespeare's Son-in-Law: John Hall, Man and Physician* (Hamden, Conn: Archon, 1964), p. 93. Joseph speculates that Mrs. Wilson was probably the vicar's wife at Stratford-on-Avon; Lapworth is mentioned in Raach's directory as practicing at Warwick, Warwickshire, some 9 miles from Stratford (p. 62).

[16]Venner, *Via recta*, "Preface".

[17]See Guidat, *Register* for the names of well-to-do clients who went to Bath. Also the *Calendar of State Papers* records the petitions of many who requested passes to travel to Bath during the time when travel was restricted. For example Vol. 12 (1658), p. 576. Sir Edward Witherington requested a pass for himself, his lady, 3 men servants and 2 maid servants. Because so many of the gentry attended the baths, they had their own "Crosse Bath" which was reserved for their use. It was this section which John Evelyn used, in 1654; see C.D. O'Malley, "John Evelyn and Medicine," *Medical History* 12 (1968):226.

[18]George Harris, "Domestic Everyday Life, Manners, and Customs in this Country, from the Earliest Period to the end of the eighteenth century," *Transactions of the Royal Historical Society* 9 (1881): 239; F.N.L. Poynter, W. J. Bishop, eds., *A Seventeenth Century Doctor and His Patients: John Symcotts 1592?-1662.* (Luton, Bedfordshire: Bedfordshire Historical Record Society Vol. 32, 1951) p. 25. For other examples of adverse travel conditions see Alice Thornton, *The Autobiography of Mrs. Alice Thornton of East Newton Co. York,* ed. D. Jackson (Durham, Andrews & Co., 1875), pp 41, 42. Somewhat later in the century, Celia Fiennes gives an excellent description of the difficulties encountered in horseback travel between 1685 and 1703 in *The Journeys of Celia Fiennes,* see especially pp. xxx-xxxii of the Introduction.

[19]Harris, "Domestic Everyday Life" p. 239.

[20]Nicholas Culpeper, *A Physical Directory or a Translation of the London Dispensatory* (London, 1649; Thomason E 576 (1) p. 49. London practitioners were not completely spared the hazards of travel; Dr. Mumford made the trip from London to Belvoir Castle in 1604, a distance of approximately 120 miles; see the *Rutland MSS* in *Reports of the Royal Commission on Historical Manuscripts* Vol. IV, p. 454. See also the case of John Evelyn and the death of his young son. J. Bowle, ed., *Diary of John Evelyn* (Oxford: Oxford University Press, 1983) pp. 94, 95.

[21]Wm. J. Bishop, "Transport and the Doctor in Great Britain," *Bulletin of the Institute of the History of Medicine* 22 (1948): 427. Bishop notes that the fee doubled.

[22]Frances P. Verney and Margaret M. Verney, eds., *Memoirs of the Verney Family* 2 vols. (London: Longmans, Green and Co., 1925), 1: p. 573.

[23]Eustace F. Bosanquet, "English Seventeenth-Century Almanacks," *The Library* Fourth Series, 10 (March, 1930): 390.

[24]Humfrey Lloyde, trans., *The Treasuri of Health* (London 1550; S.T.C. 14652), "Introduction."

[25]R. Banister, *A Treatise of one hundred and thirteene Diseases of the Eyes.* (London, 1622. Reprinted., Amsterdam: Da Capo Press, 1971) "To the Reader".

[26]*Ibid.,* "To the Reader".

[27]*Ibid.,* "To the Reader". It is noteworthy that Lincoln and Bury St. Edmonds are 125 miles apart, giving some idea of the scope of Banister's travels. For the purposes of this paper, all distances referred to are approximate. Calculations were arrived at by using modern maps and mileage aids. For an interesting seventeenth-century road guide see *Englishe Traveller: A Direction for the English Traveller* (London, 1635. Reprint ed., New York: Da Capo Press, 1969).

[28]R. Hawes, *The Poore-mans Plaster Box* (London, 1634. Reprint ed., Amsterdam: Walter J. Johnson, 1974.) See "Introduction".

[29]Hawes, p. 34.

[30]Lewis Millwater, *Cure of Ruptures in Man's Bodie. By Physical and Chirurgical Meanes and Medicines* (London, 1650; Thomason E625 (9)).

[31]A.M., *A Treatise Concerning the Plague and the Pox.* (London, 1642; Thomason E 670 (2)), in dedication "To the Reader".

[32]N. Culpeper, *Galen's Art of Physick* (London, 1652; Wing E 1287 (3)) see "Forward". On this point see also T. Vicary, *The Surgions Directorie* (London, 1651) in the chapter on women, p. 7.

[33]Richard Elkes, *Approved Medicines of Little Cost, to Preserve health and also to cure those that are sick, Provided for the souldiers Knap-Sack and the Country Man's Closet* (London, 1651; Thomason (E1370 (2)). See "Dedication".

[34]Robert Turner, trans. *The Compleat Bone Setter* (London, 1656; Thomason E 1673).

[35]John Smith, *A Compleat Practice of Physick* (London, 1656; Thomason E 1630), "Epistle to the Reader."

[36]Leonard Guthrie "The Lady Sedley's Receipt Book, 1686 and other Seventeenth Century Receipt Books," *Proceedings of the Royal Society of Medicine* (Section on British History) 6 (1913): 165.

[37]Robert Boyle *Medicinal Experiments* (London 1688) in *The Works of Robert Boyle*, 6 Vols. ed. Thomas Birch (Hildesheim: Georg Olms Verlangsbuchhandlung, 1965) 5: pp. 312-391. Boyle actually prepared medications for the use of some sufferers. See the famous case of Lady Anne Conway who suffered for most of her adult life from debilitating headaches: *Conway letters: the correspondence of Anne, Viscountess Conway, Henry More, and their friends, 1642-1684*. ed. M.H. Nicholson (Oxford: Oxford University Press, 1930) p. 225.

[38]*Ibid.*, p. 316. For an example of how a practising physician in the late seventeenth century respected Boyle's knowledge of medications, see Pierce, *Bath Memoirs*, "Preface".

[39]Plenis de Campy, Trans. E.W., *A Treatise of Phlebotomy* (London, 1658; Thomason E 1929), p. 175.

[40]Verney and Verney, *Memoirs* 1:572, 573.

[41]Ibid.

[42]Hoby, *Diary*, p. 184; see also the footnote p. 184.

[43]*Ibid.*, pp. 113-115, 147.

[44]*Ibid.*, p. 136.

[45]*Ibid.*, p. 179.

[46]Searle *Barrington Letters*, p. 20. The editor notes that Burnett received 15 payments in 5 years while Remington received 10 payments in the same period. See also Raach, *A Directory*, pp. 101-103.

[47]Searle, p. 172. In 1630, Raach shows only one qualified practitioner at Salisbury, Richard Haydocke. Possibly he was overworked and unwilling to travel 14 miles to administer "phisicke" to one young woman who seemed in good health.

[48]Dorothy Gardiner (ed.),*The Oxinden Letters 1607-1642* (London: Constable and Co. 1933). Dr. Randolph was a graduate of Oxford with an M.D. from Padua in 1626: Raach, p. 56.

[49]Verney and Verney, *Memoirs* 2:128.

[50]Ibid., *Memoirs* 2:116. This was probably Buckingham, approximately 10 miles away, still a considerable distance to travel for medical assistance.

[51]Thornton, *Autobiography*, pp. 42, 43, 132, 169-170.

[52]John Loftis (ed.), *The Memoirs of Ann, Lady Halkett and Ann, Lady Fanshawe* (Oxford: Clarendon Press, 1979), p. 33.

[53]See also Raach, p. 126; even this physician's dates are indeterminate; they are shown as 1606?-16? A further complication arises from the fact that there are two Newbiggins in Cumberland, one about 10 miles from Naworth, the other, 20-25 miles.

[54]Brilliana Harley, *The Letters of Brilliana Harley* (London: Camden Society, 1854: reprint, 1968).

[55]Raach, p. 120

[56]Harley, pp. 39-40.

[57]*Ibid.*, p. 119.

[58]Raach, p. 95.

[59]Harley, p. 91.

[60]*Ibid.*, p. 119.

[61]*Ibid.*, p. 125.

[62]*Ibid.*, p. 155.

[63]*Ibid.*, p. 127.

[64]The fact that the well-to-do Harleys were required to wait for the doctor, or in Brilliana's case do without his services, points out the hopeless situation of many people of the lower classes.

[65]Lady Ann Clifford, ed. Victoria Sackville-West, *The Diary of Lady Ann Clifford* (London: William Heinemann Ltd., 1923), p. 58.

[66]Lady Jane Bacon, *Private Correspondence of Jane, Lady Cornwallis 1613-1644* (London: S. & J. Bentley, Wilson & Fley, 1842), p. 164.

[67]*Calendar of State Papers, Domestic Series Commonwealth* 6 (1653-54) p. 9.

[68]Norman Penny, (ed.), *The Household Account Book of Sarah Fell of Swarthmoor Hall* (Cambridge: Cambridge University Press, 1920) Introduction, p. xxxii.

[69]*Ibid.*, p. 163.

[70]Raach, p. 126.

[71]Ralph Josselin, ed. Alan MacFarlane, *Diary of Ralph Josselin 1616-1683* (London: Oxford University Press, n.s., 1976), p. 50.

[72]*Ibid.*, pp. 584, 585.

[73]*Ibid.*, p. 643.

[74]John Evelyn, ed. John Bowle, *Diary of John Evelyn* (Oxford: Oxford University Press, 1983), p. 95. Dr. Jasper Needham was a graduate of Cambridge and Oxford who obtained his M.D. in 1657 and resided at Salisbury Court, see *The Memoirs of Ann Lady Fanshawe* (London: John Lane the Bodley Head, 1907), p. 586.

[75]Thornton, *Autobiography*, pp. 152, 157-158.

[76]Clifford, *Diary*, pp. 51-55. During the course of the time which the mother was alone, she had one fit which lasted "6 or 7 hours" (p. 52).

[77]W.R. Le Fanu, "A North-Riding Doctor in 1609," *History of Medicine* 5 (1961): 178. The unknown doctor was probably a surgeon who also practised physic. No licensed physician is located in this area in Raach's study. (Raach: pp. 127, 128). Moreover, the nature of his treatment (i.e. blood letting) points more to a license in surgery than a physician's training.

[78]*Calendar of State Papers, Domestic Series*, Commonwealth, Vol, 2 (1650), pp.125, 127.

[79]Joseph, *John Hall*. See the map on the frontispiece. Note that Hall's records which form *Select Observations on English Bodies* (London; 1657) are printed in Joseph. Raach's directory does not credit Hall with any degree beyond an M.A. (p. 52). However Joseph speculates that during five years of his past which are unaccounted for, he probably obtained his medical degree. (pp. 4-5).

[80]Joseph, p. 45.

[81]Hall in Joseph, pp. 54, 70.

[82]*Ibid.*, pp. 99, 159.

[83]*Ibid.*, pp. 79, 36.

[84]*Ibid.*, p. 150.

[85]Phipps practised between 1599-1637, at Kenilworth and Coventry some thirty miles from Stratford according to Raach (p. 117).

[86]Hall in Joseph, pp. 142-143.

[87]*Ibid.*, p. 163.

[88]Joseph, pp. 9, 10.

[89]Poynter and Bishop, *John Symcotts*. Raach shows Symcotts as a fully qualified

practitioner with his B.A., M.A., and M.D. (Cantab), Raach, p. 85.

[90]Poynter and Bishop, map p. 5.

[91]*Ibid.*, p. 79.

[92]*Ibid.*, pp. 79, 81, 80, 49, 82.

[93]For example, the treatment of an inflamed eye included purges, ointments and plasters for which Powers was charged £0.10.9, *Ibid.*, p. 30.

[94]*Ibid.*, p. 28.

[95]*Ibid.*, p. 30.

[96]*Ibid.*, p. 36.

[97]*Ibid.*, p. 41.

[98] *Ibid.*, p. 13.

[99]*Reports of the Royal Commission on Historical Manuscripts, Rutland MSS* Vol. 4, pp. 461, 501. The manuscripts as well as the *Dictionary of National Biography* show several spellings of the Earl of Rutland's name as well as his physician's name. Raach shows Rigesley (Ridgley), Thomas, to have been a fully qualified practitioner: B.A., M.A., M.D. (Cantab.): Raach, p. 77.

[100]Michael MacDonald, *Mystical Bedlam: Madness, Anxiety and History in Seventeenth Century England* (Cambridge: Cambridge University Press, 1981). MacDonald notes that Napier was not a qualified practitioner, but Raach has included him in his list of practitioners: Raach, p. 97. Napier cast horoscopes and read astrological signs as did other physicians of his time. He also used many of the standard treatments of the day and judged within the period in which he lived and worked, had apparently acquired some skill at diagnosis.

[101]MacDonald, p. 56.

[102]Walter Menzies, "Alexander Read, Physician and Surgeon, 1580-1641, His Life, Works, and Library," *The Library 4th Ser. 12 (1932): 48.*

[103]Raach, pp. 113,126.

[104]Menzies, p. 60. Menzies also notes that Owen Wood published a book in 1639, *An Alphabetical Book of Physicall Secrets Collected for the benefit, most especially of Householders in the Country.* The preface of this book was written by Alexander Read. There has been some speculation that Owen Wood was really Read. (pp. 60, 61).

[105]Richard Hunter and Ida MacAlpine, "The Diary of John Causabon" *Proceedings of the Huguenot Society of London* 21 (1966): 44.

[106]*Ibid.*, p. 40.

[107]*Ibid.*, p. 44.

[108]*Ibid.*, p. 44.

[109]*Ibid.*, p. 46.

[110]*Ibid.*, pp. 49, 50.

[111]*Ibid.*, p. 52.

[112]*Ibid.*, p. 53.

[113]Roger Lowe, ed. William L. Sachse, *The Diary of Roger Lowe* (New Haven: Yale University Press, 1938).

[114]See David Cressy, *Literacy and the Social Order* (Cambridge: Cambridge University Press, 1980) for the most recent study of literacy in Tudor and Stuart England. Although mercers apparently ranked quite high in literacy skills, Cressy's figures were based on the simple test of whether a respondent could merely sign his name. Roger Lowe's skills apparently went far beyond this: Cressy, p. 132.

[115]Roger accompanied his friend John Potter (who lived in Ashton), to Winnick, some 6 or 7 miles distant, when he had a bad tooth ache. Unfortunately, Corles

broke the tooth when he attempted to pull it: Lowe, p. 116.

[116]Lowe, p. 77. For another example of primitive treatment in the provinces, see John Ward's diary, where he mentioned that men in Cheshire who were sick tied handkerchiefs around their heads, and made themselves a "drink of hot milk mixed with ale or wine, sugar and spices (commonly known as a "posset"): *Diary of the Rev. John Ward* (London: Colborn, 1839), p. 175.

[117]D. C. Coleman, *The Economy of England* (Oxford: Oxford University Press, 1977) p. 11.

[118]Lowe, p. 108.

[119]Raach, *Directory*, p. 126.

[120]*Ibid.*, p. 126. Chester was approximately 22 miles from Ashton.

[121]Raach's study was used to arrive at the figure of 415 parishes. By way of comparison, see the French Monarchy's novel (but ineffective) solution to the problem of providing medical treatment for remote areas by the use of *boites de remedes du roi:* Toby Gelfand "Public Medicine and Medical Careers in France during the reign of Louis XV" *The Town and State Physician in Europe from the Middle Ages to the Enlightenment.* A. Russell, ed. (Wolfenbuttel: Herzog, August, pp. 99-123), p. 106.

Chapter II

[1]A.L. Bier, *The Problem of the Poor in Tudor and Early Stuart England*, (London: Methuen, 1983), pp. 4-7. The term "settled poor" is borrowed from this study. While 20th century studies have confirmed beyond question the link between poverty and ill health, it is noteworthy that 17th century observers were able to make the connection as well; See Thomas Cocke, *Kitchin-physick or Advice to the Poor By Way of Dialogue*, (London, 1676; Wing C4792).

[2]Margaret Pelling, "Healing the Sick Poor: Social Policy and Disability in Norwich 1550-1640," *Medical History* 29 (1985) :122; Pelling and Webster, "Medical Practitioners" pp. 225-226. For independent confirmation of the variety and number of practitioners in Norwich in 1637, see quotation by R. Burton, Norwich practitioner and author of the *Anatomy of Melancholy* in Sir George Newman, *Interpreters of Nature* (Freeport, N.Y.: Books for Libraries Press, 1968), p. 49.

[3]Pelling, "Healing the Sick Poor", p. 128; for the Norwich "Census of the poor," see p. 119.

[4]Webster, *The Great Instauration*, p. 292. For another commentary on the difficulties imposed by war, see Nellie J.M. Kerling, "A seventeenth Century Hospital Matron: Margaret Blague," *London and Middlesex Archeological Society Transactions* 22, part 3 (1979): 34-35. See also J.J. Keevil, "The Seventeenth Century English Medical Background," *Bulletin of the History of Medicine*, 31 (1957):419.

[5]Pelling, "Healing the Sick Poor," p. 126; John Patten, *English Towns 1500-1700* (Folkstone, Kent: Dawson-Archon Books, 1978), p. 42.

[6]A.B. Shaw, "Benjamin Gooch, Eighteenth-Century Norfolk Surgeon," *Medical History* 16 (1972) :40-50. Outside of London, general hospitals scarcely existed according to Delmage. See H. Levy "The Economic History of Sickness and Medical Benefit Before the Puritan Revolution," *Economic History Review*, 13 (1943) :42-57.

[7]W.K. Jordan, *Philanthropy in England 1480-1660* (London: George Allen and Unwin Ltd. 1959), p. 273.

[8]Pelling, "Healing the Sick Poor," p. 117.

[9]E.H. Phelps-Brown and Sheila V. Hopkins, "Seven Centuries of Building

Wages," *Economica* 22, 87, (1955) :205.

[10] Bier, *The Problem of the Poor*, p. 7.

[11]C. Hill, *Change and Continuity*, p. 157. See also D'Arcy Power, "The Fees of our Ancestors," *The Lancet* (Feb. 7, 1920), p. 340.

[12]Poynter and Bishop, *John Symcotts*, p.. xxvi; the editors also suggest the interesting comparison between Symcotts' fee of 2s6d and that charged by his nephew in 1684, almost 50 years later, to the wealthy Sir William Becher of Renhold. Becher paid £7.10.6 to young Symcotts and £4.13.6 to a consultant during his two week illness.

[13]Le Fanu, "North-Riding Doctor," p. 178.

[14]Hunter and McAlpine, "Diary of John Causabon," p. 49.

[15]MacDonald, *Mystical Bedlam*, p. 51.

[16]Ibid., p. 132.

[17]Private communication from Dr. J.D. Alsop: British Library, Sloane MS.1055. fo 69V, fo 76, fo 69, fo 68V.

[18]According to Phelps-Brown and Hopkins, ("Building Wages," p. 205), at this time Fleetwood would be earning approximately 18p. daily. If Fleetwood worked 5 days a week (unlikely in the building trade) he would earn 9s. a week. This medicine therefore represents a major outlay of more than 1 1/2 week's wages.

[19]Private communication from Dr. J.D. Alsop: British Library, Sloane MS 3773 (probably a west country apothecary's notebook, 1669-1674) fo 54V, fo 57, fo 61V and fo 68V.

[20]*Reports of the Royal Commission on Historical Manuscripts, Rutland MSS.* Vol. 4. pp. 454, 457, 501, 522, 540. Vol. 9, p. 393 (a) Sixth Report, p. 228 (b).

[21]Private communication from Dr. J.D. Alsop: British Library, Harley MS 1454 fo 51. This could also be evidence of overcharging, of which apothecaries were accused. See below, pp. 27, 28 this chapter.

[22]G. Roberts, ed., *Diary of Walter Yonge, Esq.* (Camden Society 1848; reprint 1968), p. xxiii. This diary was written between 1604-1628. The fees seem very high for this early in the century.

[23]Verney and Verney, *Memoirs*, 1:561.

[24]Ibid., Vol. 1:367. Sir Ralph felt he should have paid £50 but he was having financial difficulties at the time (1647). Midwives fees were, by comparison, extremely low. See also P. Chamberlen, *A Voice in Rhama*, later in this chapter.

[25]Verney and Verney, *Memoirs*, 1:574.

[26]Ibid., 1:574.

[27]Ibid., 1:434.

[28]Power, "Fees," p. 350.

[29]Poynter and Bishop, *Symcotts*, p. xxvi.

[30]David Cressy, *Literacy and the Social Order* (Cambridge: Cambridge University Press, 1980).

[31]Ibid., p. 119.

[32]See R. Carew later in the chapter.

[33]William Clowes, *A Right Frutefull and Approoved Treatise, for the Artificiall Cure of that Malady called in Latin Struma and in English, the Evill, cured by Kings and Queenes of England* (London, 1602; S.T.C. 193) "Epistle to the Reader". In 1673, Mrs. More paid 7s, 9p for medication in the hope of obtaining a cure for the "evil" (King's evil or scrofula) for her son. Private communication, Dr. J.D. Alsop, British Library, Sloane MS 3773.fo.55.

[34]Richard Hawes, *The Poor man's Plaster Box.* (London, 1634; Reprint

Amsterdam: Walter Johnson, 1974), title page.

[35]Ibid., p. 10.

[36]Ibid., pp. 11, 43.

[37]Ibid., p. 44.

[38]Alexander Read, *Most Excellent and Approved Medicines and Remedies for Most Diseases and Maladies Incident to Man's Body* (London, 1651; Thomason, E1301) "Foreword".

[39]Nicholas Culpeper, *A Physicall Directory, or , A Translation of the London Dispensatory made by the Colledge of Physicians in London* (London, 1649; Thomason, E576 1) from the "Introduction". As F.N.L. Poynter notes in "Nicholas Culpeper and His Books," *Journal of the History of Medicine* 17 (1962) :158, Culpeper was not a member of the College and was not authorized by it to make the translation. He was commissioned to make it, however, possibly by the apothecaries.

[40]N. Culpeper, *A New Method of Physick: or A Short View of Paracelsus and Galen's Practice: in 3 Treatises* (London, 1654; Thomason E1475(3)) p. 73.

[41]There is independent verification during the first half of the seventeenth century to support some of Culpeper's assertions. In addition to the information cited earlier, note the case of Elizabeth Elliott, a poor servant, who claimed to have spent more than £20 over a seven year period on a sore leg; private communication from Dr. J.D. Alsop: British Library, Sloane MS. 640 fo 350V.

[42]N. Culpeper, *Culpeper's School of Physick* (London, 1659; Thomason E 1739). "Forward", p. 29.

[43]Richard Carew, *Excellent Helps Really Found Out, tried and had (where of the Parties hereafter mentioned are true and sufficient witnesses) by a Warming Stone* (London, 1652; Thomason E 802 (1)).

[44]Thomas Brugis, *Vade Mecum or a Companion for a Chyrurgion: fitted for times of peace or war* (London, 1651: Thomason E 1357 (2)) p. 122.

[45]W. Bremer, "The Excellency of our English Bathes and the Use of them" written by D. Turner and published as part of T. Vicary *The Surgions Directorie* (London, 1651; Thomason E 1265).

[46]John Tanner, *The Hidden Treasures of the Art of Physick; Fully Discovered in Four Books* (London, 1658; Thomason E 1847), "Preface."

[47]Lancelot Coelson, *The Poor-mans Physician and Chyrurgion* (London, 1656; Thomason E 1666 (2)), "Epistle Dedicatory".

[48]Thomas Willis, *A Plain and Easie Method For Preserving [By God's Blessing] those that are Well from the Infection of the Plague, or any Contagious Distempers in City, Camp, Fleet etc. and for Curing such as are Infected with it* (London, 1666; Wing W2852).

[49]Ibid., p. 35. This is another example of how socio-economic factors influenced the perceived quality of care.

[50]Webster, *The Great Instauration*, p. 288.

[51]George Starkey, *Nature's Explication and Helmont's Vindication or a Short and Sure way to a long and Sound Life* (London, 1656; Thomason E 1635 (2)).

[52]Ibid., pp. 22, 33.

[53]Ibid., p. 164. Starkey is probably referring to diarrhoea. See above, p. 22 for independent confirmation of Starkey's allegation regarding the expense of treating diarrhoea.

[54]Ibid., p. 210.

[55]Ibid., p. 56. See John Ward, Ed. C. Severn, *Diary of the Rev. John Ward A.M: Vicar of Stratford-Upon-Avon, 1648-1679* (London: Henry Colborne, 1839) for other

evidence of possible collusion between physicians and apothecaries (p. 278).

[56]Starkey, pp. 204, 222, 224.

[57]Ibid., p. 222. Although Starkey criticizes the apothecary for his complicity in overcharging patients, he blames the doctor for arranging and enforcing the deception. Starkey claimed that some apothecaries were so upset at the situation, they had abandoned their London shops and moved to the country.

[58]Nathaniel Hodges, *Vindiciae Medicinae & Medicorum: Or an Apology For the Profession and Professors of Physic* (London, 1665; Wing H2307).

[59]Ibid., chapter 2, "Of Practising Apothecaries", pp. 49-72.

[60]Ibid., p. 39. Hodges' arguments contradicted themselves; he decried the proliferation of empirics yet demanded further restriction of licensed physicians who, in turn would be expected as "true physicians" to treat the great numbers of poor without charge!

[61]Thomas Cocke, *Kitchin-physick*. Cocke's book is of interest because he stressed diet and common sense measures in a way which was relatively foreign to his contemporaries but reminiscent of sixteenth-century writer-physician Andrew Borde who published *Here followeth a compendyous regyment or a dyetary of helth* in 1542 (S.T.C., 3379).

[62]Ibid., pp. 86, 87. While there seems to be general agreement between the various writers about the high cost of apothecaries' fees, detailed studies of not only apothecaries' accounts, but also those of the doctors who customarily used their services would be needed to arrive at an informed opinion of whether the doctor or apothecary or both were guilty of overcharging. There is evidence of some extremely wealthy apothecaries. See Fiennes, *Journeys* p. 152. See also Hunter and McAlpine, "Diary of John Causabon," p. 49 for an example of how one poor person managed to save the doctor's fee by going straight to the apothecary and "sampling" the doctor's medicine there. In 1667 William Walwyn advocated doing away with apothecaries and having physicians prepare medication, see William Walwyn, *A Touchstone for Physick* (London, 1667: Wing W693).

[63]R. Pitt in William Brockbank "Sovereign Remedies A Critical Depreciation of the 17th-Century London Pharmacopoeia," *Medical History* 8 (1964) :1-14.

[64]Brockbank, p. 12.

[65]Peter Chamberlen, *A Voice in Rhama: or the Crie of Women and Children* (London, 1646; Thomason Tracts 167). Chamberlen was as member of the London College of Physicians as well as Physician Extraordinary to the King.

[66]Ibid., (no pagination).

[67]Ward, *Diary*, p. 107.

[68]Hunter and McAlpine, "Diary of John Causabon," p. 49. It is noteworthy that at one point Causabon was imprisoned for debt.

[69]Mary Trye, *Mediatrix or the Woman Physician* (London, 1674; Wing T3174). O'Dowd's book has been described as having little practical value beyond advertising O'Dowd's medicines. See Sir Henry Thomas "The Society of Chymical Physitians" in E.A. Underwood, Ed., *Science, Medicine and History, Essays in Honour of Charles Singer*. 2 vols. (Oxford University Press: Oxford, 1953) 2, p. 61.

[70]F.N.L. Poynter, "Nicholas Culpeper and his Books," p. 156. He was also careful, as a former apothecary, to prescribe "cheap but wholesome medicines." In addition, see the analysis of Hall's and Symcotts' case records later in the chapter and Sir Charles Edward Mallett, *A History of the University of Oxford* 3 vols. (N.Y.: Longmans Green & Co. 1924-1928) 2, p. 330. Where he states that surgeons who studied at the University of Oxford were required to treat four men without charge as a graduation

requirement.

[71]John Cooke, *Unum Necessarium or the Poor Man's Case*, (London, 1647; Thomason E425 (1)) p. 41.

[72]Ibid., pp. 5, 70.

[73]Ibid., p. 41.

[74]Ibid., p. 41.

[75]Ibid., pp. 62, 63.

[76]Ibid., pp. 64, 65.

[77]For the role of gentlewomen, see chapter five, below.

[78]Banister, *A Treatise*, "To the Reader". See also T. Vicary *The Surgions Directorie*, (London, 1651: Thomason E1265) "Dedication" on this point.

[79]Banister, p. 4.

[80]Poynter and Bishop, *John Symcotts*. In making some of these distinctions, (and taken in the context of the seventeenth century) where a patient was designated by the title of Master or Mistress, some independence of livelihood was assumed -- See OED sub "master", sub "mistress." Three children who could not be identified were not included in the calculations.

[81]The "poor woman of Fenton" for whom Symcotts prescribed.

[82]Joseph, *John Hall*, p. 73; Hall in Joseph, p. 82. In addition, six children could not be identified and were not included in the figures. Attention should also be drawn to the high proportion of females in Hall's practice, a trend which is also evident in twentieth century medical practices; Hall identified 107 females and 69 males. In *Mystical Bedlam*, MacDonald analyzed the patients with mental disorders who resorted to Napier's services and found that for every 100 females, there were only 58.2 males (p. 40).

[83]Harley, *Letters*, p. 117. The "ague", the principle symptom of which was intermittent fever, was the second most common cause of death according to John Graunt; see *Natural and Political observations made upon the bills of mortality*, ed. Walter Willcox, (Baltimore, 1939). This work was first published in 1662.

[84]Harley, *Letters*, p. 117.

[85]Hunter and McAlpine, "Diary of John Causabon", p. 43.

[86]Ibid., p. 50.

[87]Josselin, *Diary*, p 40.

[88]Ibid., p. 103. When Josselin accepted the appointment as vicar of Earles Colne in 1640, he was promised £40 in tithes which was to make up 50% of his total salary. (p. 10).

[89]Ibid., pp. 136, 221, 225.

[90]Ibid., p. 163.

[91]By 1656, Josselin was able to give his sister Anna the gift of a sum of money (in addition to a loan) and in 1657 bought his first silver plate as a gift for his children. (pp. 370, 419). By March 1658 he noted in his diary that all his debts were paid and he had an estate which he reckoned at £600. (p.421).

[92]Ibid., pp. 584, 595, 634, 642, 643. Josselin complained about the high price of medicine from the apothecary who filled the London physician's receipts.

[93]Ibid., p. 392.

[94]Searle, *Barrington Letters*, p. 114.

[95]Gardiner, *Oxinden Letters*, p. 181.

[96]See A. Read, *Most Excellent and Approved Medicines*, "Forward"; Culpeper, *Galen's Art of Physick*, (London, 1652; Thomason E1287 (3)) "To the Reader," also Culpeper *A Physicall Directory* "Introduction"; Starkey, *Natures Explication*, p. 165

speaks of the "ruines of several persons and families".

[97]Verney and Verney, *Memoirs* 1:568.

[98]Ward, *Diary*, p. 108.

[99]Verney and Verney, *Memoirs* 2:177.

[100]Ibid., 1:576.

[101]Chamberlen, *A Voice in Rhama*.

[102]George Roberts, (ed.), *Diary of Walter Yonge Esq. 1604-1628* (London, Camden Society, 1848; Reprint, N.Y.: Johnson Reprint Corporation, 1968) p. xxiii.

[103]Hunter and McAlpine, "Diary of John Causabon," p. 49.

Chapter III

[1]See for example Lady Jane Cornwallis, *Private Correspondence of Jane Lady Cornwallis 1613-44*, (London: S. & J. Bentley, Wilson and Hey, 1842); Lady Margaret Hoby (1570-1633) *Diary*; Josselin, *Diary*; Lady Brilliana Harley, *Letters*; F.W. Bennett, "The Diary of Isabella, Wife of Sir Roger Twysden, Baronet, of Royden Hall, East Peckham, 1645-1651," *Archaeologia Cantiana* 41 (1939) pp. 113-136. One study by P. Laslett and John Harrison concluded that in 1688 "no less than 28% of children in Clayworth came from homes broken by death." See "Clayworth and Cogenhoe" in H. Bell and R. Ollard eds. *Historical Essays 1600-1750*, (London: Adam and Charles Black, 1963) pp. 157-184.

[2]Judith Simmons, "Publications of 1623," *The Library* 5th series, 21 (1966): pp. 207-222.

[3]For an example of how two children viewed the correlation between their "sins" and the death of a parent, see Oliver Heywood, E. Axon (ed), *Life of John Angier* (Manchester, for the Chetham Society: 1937, Reprint, Johnson Reprint Corporation, 1968) p. 126.

[4]Edward Burghall, T.W. Barlow (ed), *Diary of the Rev. Edward Burghall, Vicar of Acton, Chester 1628-1663* or *Providence Improved* (Manchester: John Gray Bell, 1855).

[5]Ibid., p. 157.

[6]Ibid., p. 153.

[7]Robert Wright, *A Receyt to Stay the Plague; delivered in a Sermon* (London 1625; S.T.C. 26037) pp. 22-23. See also I. Vincent, *God's Terrible Voice in the City, Two late dreadful judgements of Plague and Fire in London* (London 1667; Wing V440). Vincent urged repentance to prevent further outbreaks of the plague.

[8]Josselin, *Diary* p. 519. Josselin's diary contains numerous references to days of "public humiliacion" in his parish. He noted in his diary that on July 16, 1665, 1268 plague victims had been buried and another 725 were infected, moving him to pray "Lord hold thy hand". Note also Blair Worden, "Providence and politics in Cromwellian England," *Past and Present*, 109 (1985): 55-99 (p. 70).

[9]Thomas Mayerne in Cook, "The Regulation of Medical Practice" p. 131.

[10]William Boraston in William Bremer, *The Englishman's Treasure*, 9th ed. (London: 1641; Wing V334). This edition contained sections by Thomas Vicary, William Turner and W.B. (probably William Boraston).

[11]Robert Bayfield, *Enchiridion Medicum: Containing the Causes, Signs and Cures of all those Diseases that do chiefly affect the body of Man* (London, 1655; Thomason E1563) p. 320.

[12]Samuel Hartlib, *A Table of Chymical, Medical and Chirurgical Addresses made to Samuel Hartlib Esq.* (London 1655; Thomason E1509 (2)).

[13]Cooke, *Kitchin-Physick* p.33. For the strongly religious views of a puritan physician at the end of the century see Peter Krivatsky, "William Westmacott's Memorabilia: The Education of a Puritan Country Physician," *Bulletin of the History of Medicine* 49 (1975): 331-338.

[14]Josselin, *Diary* pp. 32, 33. See also pp. 36, 72 for examples of how Josselin saw a direct relationship between good health, ill health and providence. Brilliana Harley also saw illness as a correction. See Harley, *Letters* p. 44.

[15]Josselin, p. 14. A quotidian ague was a fever which recurred daily. (OED)

[16]Ibid., p. 415.

[17]Ibid., pp. 111, 403, 215. Josselin felt that his wife had "saved a woman's life" in childbirth, possibly by prayer. See also Mary Rich, Countess of Warwick, *Autobiography* p. 216. Lady Warwick (the sister of Robert Boyle) stayed all night praying at the delivery of Ann Barrington.

[18]Josselin, p. 510.

[19]Ibid., p. 572.

[20]Marjorie Hope Nicholson, *Conway Letters: the correspondence of Anne, Viscountess Conway, Henry More, and their friends, 1642-1684.* (Oxford: Oxford University Press, 1930). An excellent account of Greatrakes, his attempted cure of Lady Conway's crippling headaches and his successful cure of many others can be found in Nicholson's volume, pp. 244-308. For other examples of well-intentioned healers who used methods similar to Greatrakes, at no charge, see Keith Thomas, *Religion and the Decline of Magic* (New York: Charles Scribner & Sons, 1971), pp. 201, 202.

[21]Lewis Millwater, *The Cure of Ruptures in Man's Bodies* (London, 1650; Thomason E625 (a)) no pagination. For a doctor's argument against faith healing or miraculous cures see John Cotta, *A Short Discoverie*, p. 36.

[22]For a full description of seventeenth-century healing by touch, see Thomas, *Religion and the Decline of Magic*, pp. 192-204.

[23]Webster, *The Great Instauration*, p. 255.

[24]Phyllis Allen, "Medical Education in 17th Century England," *Journal of History of Medicine* I(1946): 115-143.

[25]Ibid., p. 142.

[26]F.E. Halliday, "Sir Richard Carewes Booke'," *Practitioner* 176 (1956): 54; Keith Thomas, *Religion and the Decline of Magic*, p. 275. Thomas notes that because Atwell's cures worked, he was suspected of practising magic.

[27]Josselin, *Diary*, p. 221.

[28]Ibid., p. 402. Evidently the minister died 8 days after the man bit him.

[29]Poynter and Bishop, *Symcotts*, p. 52.

[30]John Rogers, Ed. E. Rogers *Some Account of the Life and Opinions of John Rogers* (London: Longmans Green, 1867).

[31]John Ward, *Diary*, p. 117.

[32]F.J. Powicke, *A Life of the Reverend Richard Baxter*, 2 vols. (London: Jonathan Cape, 1924-27) 1:104, 105. Baxter said that he was treated by more than 36 doctors in his youth, all of whom "made matters worse." p. 87

[33]Ibid., pp. 104, 105. For an example of a woman who used her healing skills to proseletyze, see Hanlon, (Sister Joseph Damien), "These Be But Women," in Charles H. Carter, ed., *From the Renaissance to the Counter Reformation* (New York: Random House, 1965) p. 379.

[34]Roger Lowe, *Diary*, pp. 17, 18. Perhaps Roger took the time to copy the lengthy receit into his diary because of his tendency to overindulge in alcoholic beverages.

[35]Cotta, *A Short Discoverie*. According to Raach, Cotta was a fully qualified physician with his B.A., M.A., and M.D. degrees from Cambridge. (Raach, p. 38).

[36]Ibid., pp. 88, 89.

[37]Ibid, p. 84.

[38]Ibid., pp. 87, 88.

[39]Ibid., pp. 90-93. To support his charge, Cotta cited two instances, where, he claimed , patients were making a good recovery under a physician's care and were persuaded to switch their allegiance to a parson - physician (Cotta's term), which greatly retarded their progress.

[40]James Primrose, Trans. Robert Wittie, *Popular Errours or the Errours of the People in Physick* (London, 1651; Thomason E1227). Originally written in Latin, this treatise was, like Cotta's, highly critical of all medical practitioners other than qualified physicians.

[41]See also Edmund Gayton, *The Religion of a Physician*, (London, 1663; Wing G416). Gayton presents the opposite side of the coin where the physician undertakes a spiritual as well as physical role as healer stating: "The Physick of the body is but a preparative for the bettering of the Soul...." (Forward)

[42]As an illustration of this traditional assistance, we may note the 1611 will of Sir Francis Carew of Beddington, Surrey. Carew left legacies to the cleric, Daniel Meede, for his aid rendered during Carew's illness, and to an apothecary, but made no reference to a physician or surgeon. E. Stokes, "Surrey Wills Proved in the Prerogative Court of Canterbury in 1611," *Surrey Archeological Collections, 35 (1924), p. 39.*

[43]Thomas, *Religion and the Decline of Magic*, 278. See also Josselin, *Diary* for examples of self treatment augmented by faith and prayer. (pp. 40, 17, 218, 447, 191, 186).

[44]Warwick, *Autobiography*. See also *The Diary of Lady Margaret Hoby* for another gentlewoman who augmented her healing skills with prayer.

[45]Warwick, p. 99.

[46]Ibid., p. 148. Lady Warwick also described the death of the young Duke of Kendal in 1667 of convulsive fits; four doctors were unable to save him. The implication is that they should have bent their efforts toward ensuring his soul's well-being.

[47]Ibid., pp. 153, 157, 182, 207.

[48]Ibid., p. 29.

[49]Robert Boyle, *Robert Boyle The Works*, 4, p. 39.

[50]Ibid., p. 41. Boyle's interest in chemistry led him to the compounding of medical prescriptions. One of his clients was Lady Anne Conway, see: *Conway Letters*, p. 225.

[51]Clowes, *Artificial Cure of Struma*, "Epistle to the Reader." The type of medical literature under discussion here is not of the same calibre or genre as the highly personal and introspective work by Thomas Browne, *Religio Medici*, first published in 1642 (London). It became one of the most widely read books of its time. See C.W. Schoneveld, "Sir Thomas Browne and Leiden University, 1633," *English Language Notes* 19 (June 1982): 335-359. Schoneveld has described the work as "designed to reveal a young man's cosmopolitan response to the world" (p. 324).

[52]Cotta, *A Short Discoverie*, p. 120. The physician and surgeon as "artist" is a recurring theme. See also T. Brugis, *Vade Mecum or a Companion for a Chyrurgion: fitted for times of peace or War*. (London, 1651; Thomason E1357 (2)).

[53]Banister, *A Treatise*, see title page.

[54]Read, *Most Excellent and Approved Medicines.* Ecclesiasticus 38:, 1,2,4. In Read, title page.

[55]Ibid., "Forward." In 1626, the Countess of Bedford agreed to treatment by Dr. Theodore Mayerne. Although she did not think it would be efficacious, she felt it would be wrong not to avail herself of any means which might restore her health (Cornwallis, *Correspondence*, p. 146).

[56]Thomas Brugis, *Vade Mecum* Brugis in particular uses the artist allegory throughout his lengthy Preface, finally bringing the two themes of Art and the Divine together in the phrase "The Divine Art of Healing". Although he calls himself "Doctor in Physick," he is obviously a surgeon.

[57]Peter Levens, *The Pathway to Health* (London, 1654; Thomason E1472) Title page.

[58]This and the following quotation are from a private communication from Dr. J.D. Alsop, citing British Library, Sloane MS 236, fos. 2, 2v.

[59]The book of Ecclesiasticus was part of the Greek Bible which was intended for the Jews of the Dispersion. It is not a part of the Jewish canon from which the King James version was adopted. Ecclesiasticus is included in the Douay version which was published by the English College in 1609 at Douay and in the Jerusalem Bible which was adopted from the French version of the Old Testament. See *The Jerusalem Bible*, ed. Alexander Jones (Garden City, N.Y.: Doubleday and company Inc. 1966) "Introduction to Ecclesiasticus," pp. 1034-1035.

[60]George Stanhope, *Meditations and Prayers for Sick Persons*, 2nd ed. (London, 1700; Wing T947). Stanhope published 12 works between 1691-1699. The date when this treatise was first published in unknown, but was likely in the last decade of the seventeenth century. See also Edward Wolley, *Euroxia. A Model of Private Prayers* (London, 1661; Thomason E2130 (2)): 55-7. Wolley was a chaplain to Charles II; the prayer illustrates the general theme of sickness as God's corrective.

[61]In support of this conclusion see Paul S. Seaver, *Wallington's World* (Stanford, California: Stanford University Press, 1985). Seaver concluded that the puritan Nehemiah Wallington, a seventeenth-century London artisan "clearly regarded doctors and apothecaries as a last desperate measure, a predictable expense for no predictable benefit." (p. 228).

Chapter IV

[1]Joseph, *John Hall*, p. 24. Symcotts also preferred medicinal forms of treatment (especially vomits) to venesection. Surprisingly, John Causabon, the surgeon, was also uncomfortable with the procedure; See Hunter and McAlpine, "The Diary of John Causabon," pp. 38, 49, 50.

[2]Hall in Joseph, p. 18.

[3]Ibid., p. 23. Hartshorn was obtained from the antler of a hart and was a chief source of ammonia (OED).

[4]Ibid., p. 31.

[5]Guthrie, "The lady Sedley's Receipt Book," pp. 153, 154.

[6]Robert T. Gunther, ed., *The Greek Herbal of Dioscorides* (Oxford: The University Press, 1934); p. 383.

[7]Hall in Joseph, p.40.

[8]Ibid., p. 47.

[9]Ibid., p.55. An electuary was a medicine consisting of a powder or other

ingredients mixed with honey, jams or syrup (OED).

[10]Joseph, *John Hall*, p. 25. For a good example of Hall's prescriptions for scurvy, see Hall in Joseph, pp. 2, 3.

[11]Guthrie, "The Lady Sedley's Receipt Book," p. 154.

[12]R.G. Alexander, *A Plain Plantain* (Ditchling, Sussex: S. Dominic's Press, 1922); pp. 48, 49.

[13]Banister, *A Treatise*, no pagination.

[14]Poynter and Bishop, *Symcotts*, pp. 187, 188.

[15]Ibid., pp. 96, 97.

[16]J. Stevens Cox, ed., "Dorset Folk Remedies of the Seventeenth and Eighteenth centuries," *The Dorset Natural History and Archeological Society* (1962), pp. 8, 9.

[17]Poynter and Bishop, *Symcotts*, p. XII. Starkey also made this point in a different way, see Starkey, *Natures Explication*, pp. 138, 140. For another example of a man who treated himself for gout by using milk and crushed elder leaves, see Martin Blockwick, *Anatomia Sambuci* or *The Anatomie of the Elder* (London, 1655; Thomason E1534 (2)). For other cures for gout, see p. 47 this chapter.

[18]W.R. LeFanu, "A North Riding Doctor in 1609," *Journal of Medical History* 1965: 20, pp. 213-225. Senna was the dried leaflets of various species of the shrub Cassia used as a cathartic or emetic (OED).

[19]The works which were examined were arbitrarily determined; they were all of those listed under the topic "Medical Works" in *Catalogue of the Pamphlets, Books, Newspapers and Manuscripts Relating to the Civil War, The Commonwealth and Restoration, Collected by George Thomason 1640-1641* London; 1908 Vol II pp. 639, 640. Although these tracts deal with the period 1640-1660, the same type of evidence is available for the early part of the seventeenth century, that is, medical treatises, written by medical practitioners, and available to the population at large for use by lay practitioners or in self-treatment. See for example Christopher Langton, *An introduction to physicke, with an universal dyet* London, 1550(?) S.T.C 81; Humfrey Lloyde (trans.) *The Treasure of Helth contaynynge many profytable medicines gathered by Petrus Hispanus* London, 1550(?) STC 81. The latter is a very comprehensive compendium of diseases, their causes, symptoms and remedies; John Woodall, *The Surgions Mate* London, 1617 STC 946. A. Pare *Three and Fifty Instruments of Chirurgery* London, 1631 - Reprint Amsterdam & New York: Da Capo 1969. Walter Bruell *Praxis Medicinae or The Physicians Practice: Wherein are contained all inward diseases from the Head to the Foot* (London 1639 (1st edition published in 1632) STC 704) Bruell stated explicitly that his work was published not only for physicians, surgeons and apothecaries, but for "all such which are careful of their health and welfare": "Forward".

[20]Ralph Williams, *Physical Rarities containing The Most Choice Receipts of Physick and Chyrurgerie For the Cure of all Diseases incident to Man's Body* (London, 1651; Thomason E1302) pp. 175, 177, 207, 126.

[21]Ibid., p. 128.

[22]Robert Bayfield, *Enchiridion Medicum: Containing the Causes, Signs and Cures of all those Diseases, that do chiefly affect the body of man* (London, 1655; Thomason E1563) "Forward". Although Bayfield does not claim to be a physician or surgeon, he uses Greek and Latin in the treatise and the final section contains some descriptions in Latin although the bulk of his treatments are described in English - see below.

[23]Ibid., p. 320.

[24]Ibid., pp. 41, 58. Although this prescription is given in Latin, it does not disguise the fact that it is made up of ingredients in everyday use by lay people. Also noteworthy

is the non-specific nature of the prescriptions. For a good example of how educated people used non-specific medications, see Marjorie H. Nicholson, *Conway Letters* (Oxford: University Press, 1930), pp. 389-400.

[25]Francis Glisson, George Bate and Ahasuerus Regemorter, *A Treatise of the Rickets Being a Disease Common to Children* (London, 1650; Thomason E1267). Five other Fellows of the College also contributed papers which were originally published in Latin.

[26]Robert G. Frank Jr., "The Physician as Virtuoso in Seventeenth Century England," in B. Shapiro and R. Frank eds,. *English Virtuosi in the 16th and 17th Centuries* (Los Angeles: 1979, University of California Press), p. 85.

[27]Ibid., p. 332, emphasis mine.

[28]Ibid., pp. 366, 322, 368.

[29]Webster has also commented on the way that mid-seventeenth century doctors indulged in experiments in anatomy and physiology without recognizing their "medical implications", virtually regarding the new discoveries as "intellectual diversions" completely detached from the Galenic theory upon which their bread and butter depended. See Webster, *The Great Instauration*, p.. 316. See also p. 49 below.

[30]Robert Pemel, *Tractatus, De facultatibus Simplicium, The Second Part of the Nature and Qualitie of Such Physical Simples as are most frequently used in medicines* (London 1653. Thomason; E721 (2)). While this tract was directed to both laymen and professionals, Pemel, who was evidently a qualified practitioner, had written an earlier treatise which appeared to be for lay use only. See the above title omitting "The Second Part", London 1652, Thomason E660 (8), which is an example of the lack of differentiation between literature intended for popular and licensed practitioners. Martin Blockwich, *Anatomie of the Elder*, described himself as a physician-in-ordinary.

[31]Culpeper's widow claimed that he wrote 79 books. See F.N.L. Poynter, "Nicholas Culpeper and his books," p. 160.

[32]John Tanner, *The Hidden Treasure of the Art of Physick* (London, 1658; Thomason E1847); James Cooke *Mellificium Chirurgiae or the Marrow* (London, 1648; Wing C6012).

[33]Philiatros, *Nature Exenterata: or Nature Unbowelled By the Most Exquisite Anatomizer of Her* (London, 1655; Thomason E1560).

[34]W.M., *The Queen's Closet opened. Incomparable secrets in Physick, Chirurgery, Preserving, Candying and Cookery* (London, 1655; Thomason E1519). W.M. was probably a clerk or secretary to the Queen as he mentioned having personally "copied" most of the receipts. It is highly unlikely that the Queen carried out much home medical treatment considering the fees which were paid to the Royal physicians, surgeons and apothecaries. In October 1618, more than £225 was paid to the foregoing in *Reports of the Royal Commission on Historical Manuscripts. Rutland MSS 9* (2) 425b. See also the salaries of Dr. Mayerne and Dr. Colladon for the year 1655— Mayerne £200, Colladon £100 in *Calendar of State Papers, Domestic Series, Commonwealth.* 8 (1655) p. 114.

[35]In the last category was one contributor known by the initials A.R.C., one Adrian Gilbert and "the old lady of Oxford". It is interesting to note the high number of male lay practitioners in these two books in the face of the evidence that women practised medicine in upper class families rather than men. If the authors were trying

to use social status in order to promote sales of their books, as in any patriarchal society, the male head of the family unit would command the greatest prestige and recognition. In some cases, therefore, family receipts may have been designated by the name of the household head. An alternative explanation, of course, would be that there were far more male practitioners of popular medicine than has been hitherto demonstrated.

[36]Philiatros, pp. 20, 35, 2, 168, 171, 172, 334.

[37]Ibid., p.. 334.

[38]W.M., p. 140; Philiatros, pp. 168, 2.

[39]W.M., p. 156; Philiatros, p. 20.

[40]Philiatros, p. 35; W.M., p. 149.

[41]W.M., p. 126.

[42]W.M., pp. 182; Philiatros, p. 67.

[43]W.M., pp. 31, 32; Philiatros, pp. 80-81.

[44]William Brockbank, "Sovereign Remedies: A critical depreciation of the 17th-Century London Pharmacopoeia," *Medical History* 8 (1964): 9.

[45]Two other medical compendia with popular appeal were J. White, *A Rich Cabinet with Variety of Inventions* (London, 1651; Thomason E1295 (2)); Thomas Lupton, *A Thousand Notable Things of Sundry Sorts, enlarged* (London, 1659; Thomason E1747). The latter is a delightful mish-mash of information on a wide variety of topics. It contains excellent directions for setting and splinting broken bones, among other things.

[46]Samuel Boulton, *Medicina Magica Tamen Physica: Magical but Natural Physick*, (London, 1656; Thomason E1678 (2)).

[47]John Schroder (Dr. of Physick) *ZOOVTIA* or *The History of Animals as they are useful in Physick and Chirurgery* (London, 1658; Thomason E1759 (1)). See also William Williams, *Occult Physick or The three principles in Nature Anatomized by a Philosophical operation* (London, 1660; Thomason E1737 (2)). Williams divides his book into three sections, the third dealing with astrology including a tract showing the effect of the moon on a patient's urine.

[48]Brockbank, "Sovereign Remedies", p. 4.

[49]Ibid., pp. 8-9. Although Robert Frank is highly laudatory of the intellectual pursuits of the founders of "scientific" medicine, he fails to establish a link between these pursuits and their clinical application: see Frank "The Physician as Virtuoso."

[50]Edward Rosen, "Kepler's Attitude toward Astrology and Mysticism", pp. 253-273 (p. 253), Richard Westfall, "Newton and Alchemy", pp. 315-337 (p. 315) and M. Feingold "Occult Tradition at English Universities", pp. 73-89 (p. 73), all in *Occult and Scientific Mentalities in the Renaissance*, ed. B. Vickers (Cambridge: Cambridge University Press, 1984).

[51]Willis in Brockbank, p. 8.

[52]For insights into the acknowledged mentor of seventeenth-century chemical physicians, see Allen G. Debus "Some Comments on the Contemporary Helmontian Renaissance", *Ambix* 19 (1972): 145-150; Debus, *The English Paracelsians* (London: Oldbourne, 1965); Walter Pagel "Von Helmont's Concept of Disease: To be or not to be? The Influence of Paracelsus", *Bulletin of the History of Medicine* 46, no. 5 (1972): 49.

[53]This is a personal insight which has been bolstered by recent research. See A. Wear, R. French, and I. Lone, eds. *The Medical Renaissance of the Sixteenth Century* (Cambridge: Cambridge University Press, 1985) p. xv.

[54]Thomas O'Dowd in Sir Henry Thomas "The Society of Chymical Physitians an echo of the Great Plague of London, 1665" in E.A. Underwood ed. *Science, Medicine and History* 2 Vols. (London: Oxford University Press, 1953) 2, p. 50.

[55]George Thomson, *Galeno-pale or a Chymicall Trial of the Galenists, That their dross in Physick may be discovered with the grand Abuses and Disrepute they have brought upon the whole Art of Physick and Chirurgery, in their method touching Phlebotomy and Purgation* (London, 1665; Wing T1023), p. 100. What Thomson treated was a fecal impaction for which an enema would have been the most effective treatment. See also the debate between Dr. W. Simpson (chemical physician) and Dr. R. Wittie, (traditional physician) in Poynter, F.N.L. "A Seventeenth-Century Medical Controversy Robert Witty versus William Simpson" in E.A. Underwood ed. *Science Medicine and History* 2, pp. 72-81.

[56]Starkey, *Nature's Explication*, p. 30.

[57]Ibid., p. 228. Starkey's arguments at many points bear a striking similarity to those of Ivan Illich, the 20th century scholar and critic of the medical profession. See *Limits to Medicine: medical nemesis, the expropriation of health* (Harmondsworth and New York: Penguin, 1977).

[58]One of the main differences which appears to have remained an issue was that of phlebotomy. However, since many Galenists apparently made little use of bleeding, this difference was minimized. For an example of a dispute between two doctors, both apparently traditional (Galenical) practitioners, see Alice Thornton, *Autobiography*, p. 33. In this case, the patient made the final decision "...if they would save my life, I must bleed".

[59]Will Thrasher, *The Marrow of Chymical Physick or the Practice of Making Chymical Medicines* (London, 1679; Wing T1080). For an early apologia for chemical medicine based on philosphical and religious ground see Joseph Duchesne. (Trans. T. Timme) *The Practise of Chymicall and hermeticall physick* (London, 1605; S.T.C. 988). Other examples of "common" cures are found in George Phaedro (Trans. J. Andreas) *Physicall and chemicall Practise* (London, 1654; Thomason E1472 (2)) pp. 2, 30.

[60]Noah Biggs, *Mataeo Technia Medicinae Praxeos or Vanity of the Craft of Physick* (London, 1651; Thomason E625 (17)). "Forward."

[61]Ibid., "Forward". The defence of chemical medicine was not exclusively associated with a few radicals who were anti-establishment. Dr. Walter Charleton was a King's physician and in 1689, 1690 and 1691 the president of the College of Physicians. He translated several of Von Helmont's works and published them; see Charleton, *Deliramenti Catarrhi* (London, 1650; Thomason E601 (6)).

[62]*Semeiotica Uranica or An Astrological Judgement of Diseases* (London, 1651; Thomason E1360 (2)); 3rd ed. London, 1658; Thomason E1726 (London, (1)). Since Culpeper wrote for the lay public, his interest in astrology must be considered significant in any discussion of popular medicine.

[63]Christopher Heydon, *Astrological Book* (London, 1650; Thomason E1299 (3)), "Forward."

[64]Simon Forman, ed., J. Halliwell, *The Autobiography and Personal Diary of Dr. Simon Forman, the Celebrated Astrologer, From A.D. 1552 to A.D. 1602* (London: Richards Printer, 1849), pp. 15-32.

[65]MacDonald, *Mystical Bedlam*, p. 32.

[66]Elias Ashmole, *Elias Ashmole Autobiographical and Historical Notes* 5 Vol. (Oxford: Clarendon Press, 1966) 2 (1617-1660): 580. Other examples of self-treatment are on pp. 393, 451, 453.

[67]Ibid., pp. 670, 672. Ashmole received a bishop's license to practice physick in the province of Canterbury in 1670 after which he noted he began to practice "more openly and with good success" (p. 173). See below for comment by H. Dick re astrology and the surreptitious practice of medicine.

[68]R. Turner, *Paracelsus of the Supreme mysteries of Nature of the Spirits of the Planets and Occult Philosophy*, (London, 1655; Thomason E1567 (2)).

[69]See above, pp. 30, 31 for a discussion of Trigg and his work.

[70]Genevieve Miller "A Seventeenth-Century Astrological Diagnosis," in E.A. Underwood, *Science, Medicine and History*, p. 32. The example she gives is William Salmon's *Synopsis Medicinae, a Compendium of Physick, Chirurgery and Anatomy in IV Books . . . Perform'd Astrologically, Galenically and Chymically*, second ed., (London, 1681). See also William Williams, *Occult Physick*, (London, 1660; Thomason E1737 (2)).

[71]Hugh Dick "Students of physic and astrological medicine in the Age of Science," *Journal of History of Medicine and Allied Sciences*, 1, no. 3 (1946): 432. This is an excellent account of astrological medicine in the seventeenth century.

[72]Robert Boyle was one of the opponents of astrological medicine on religious grounds. For a discussion of his views see J.R. Jacobs "Robert Boyle and Subversive Religion in the Early Restoration," *Albion* VI, (1974):275-293.

[73]Eustace F. Bosanquet, "English Seventeenth-Century Almanacks," *The Library*, X (March, 1930): 365, 366.

[74]G. Naworth, *A New Almanack and Progostication for the yeare of our Lord and Saviour Jesus Christ 1644* (Oxford 1644; Thomason E118 (4)) no pagination.

[75]J. Pont, *A Generall Almanack for every yeare* (London, 1646; Thomason E1171 (1)) pp. 33, 66.

[76]Ibid., p. 67.

[77]George Wharton, *A New Almanack*, (London 1648; Thomason E1198 (2)).

[78]Bosanquet, p. 386. See also Bosanquet p. 380 for an example of an anatomical chart showing how the zodiac signs govern different parts of the body.

[79]See Cressy, *Literacy and the Social Order*. Cressy concluded that there was an increase in the number of literate Englishmen in the seventeenth century. He states, moreover, that "medical and meteorological advice of the sort found in almanacks, all put valuable information into the hands of people who could profit from it." (p. 7). What he fails to acknowledge is that those who could possibly profit the most from it were those who were illiterate.

[80]Peter Burke, *Popular Culture in Early Modern Europe* (London: Temple Smith, 1978) p. 273; C. V. Schonveld, "Sir Thomas Browne", *English Language Notes* (June, 1982) p. 330.

[81]John Smith, *A Compleat Practice of Physick* (London, 1656; Thomason E1630) p. 328.

[82]Boyle, *The Works* 5, p. 363.

[83]Starkey, *Nature's Explication*, p. 31.

[84]Pelling and Webster have reached similar conclusions in their study of sixteenth-century medical practitioners. See Pelling and Webster *Medical Practitioners*, p. 235.

Chapter V

[1]E. Joyce Cockram, for example in a "tribute" to women practitioners used the following juxtaposition "... whole districts would depend on the ministrations of the Lady of the Manor or upon travelling quacks or herb women" (p. 90). E. Joyce Cockram, "Tribute to Sabine," *Journal of the Medical Womens Federation*, July

(1961): 86-97.

[2]For a commentary on the position of sixteenth-century widows, see Pelling and Webster, "Medical Practitioners," p. 222. See also George C. Peachey, *The Life of William Savory (Surgeon), of Brightwalton,* (London: J.J. Keliher and Co. Limited, 1903) for several examples of eighteenth-century surgeon's widows who carried on their husband's practices. For a brief observation on the relative restrictions of Surgeons' and Apothecaries' guilds regarding women, see A. Clark, *Working Life,* pp. 260, 261.

[3]Margaret C. Barnet, "The Barber Surgeons of York," *Medical History* 12 (1968), p. 27. Pelling and Webster "Medical Practitioners," p. 222. For a comparison with the widows of barber-surgeons in sixteenth-century France, see Natalie Zemon Davis "Women in the Crafts in Sixteenth-Century Lyon" *Feminist Studies* 8 (1982): 46-80 (pp. 69, 70).

[4]Private communication from Dr. J.D. Alsop citing Public Record Office, London, MS E179/251/22.

[5]Sidney Young, *The Annals of the Barber Surgeons of London,* p. 270.

[6]Ibid., pp. 264, 268, 270.

[7]J. Elise Gordon, "Some Women Practitioners of Past Centuries," *Practitioner* 208 (1972): 566-80.

[8]Searle, *Barrington Letters,* p. 191.

[9]Pelling, "Occupational Diversity," p. 509.

[10]Pelling and Webster, "Medical Practitioners," p. 233.

[11]Josselin, *Diary,* p. 468. Mrs. Withers obtained good results in both cases.

[12]Clark, *Royal College of Physicians.*

[13]Raach, *A Directory,* p. 14.

[14]See Chapter 2 above on this point. In addition, using Raach's own figures, there was only one doctor in the whole of the county of Cumberland who practised for only 8 of the 37 years covered by the study (p. 126). Even for the Midlands, Raach acknowledges only one doctor within the county of Rutland (p. 113). Clearly Raach's statement is too sweeping to account for the regional and social limitations of professional health care in this period.

[15]Ibid., p. 50.

[16]Ibid, p. 74. It is likely that Prudence Potter's tombstone in the church yard of Newton St. Petrock, N. Devon is the only known surviving source to establish her identity and skill. It described her thus: "Her life was spent in the industrious, charitable and successful practice of medicine, chirurgery and midwifery," See a letter from Dr. Nesbitt Burns, "A woman doctor of the 17th century," *British Medical Journal,* 1(1941): 124.

[17]The two local studies which Raach consulted to supplement his analysis of bishops' records, wills, university records and a few scattered sources were "Devon Medical Worthies," in *Devon and Cornwall Notes and Queries,* Series 13 (1925) and 14 (1926) and "Cambridgeshire Doctors in the Olden Times" in the *Proceedings of the Cambridge Antiquarian Society* 15 (1911). In his Introduction, Raach does not mention the imbalance of sexes in his study or try to account for it; there is also no comment on the two women who were included.

[18]Pelling, "Occupational Diversity," pp. 489, 508. See also Pelling, "A Survey of East Anglian Medical Practitioners 1500-1640," *Local Population Studies* 25 (1980): 54-55 for her assessment of Raach's work in which she notes that Raach failed to "take into account other classes of practitioners and accepted academically qualified practitioners at their own valuation." (p. 54).

[19]Raach included the name of Bauer, which was mentioned by Brilliana Harley, see Harley, *Letters*, p. 119. He failed to include female practitioners such as those mentioned in Walter Yonge *Diary*, p. xxii, or Searle, *Barrington Letters*, p. 191, or Verney and Verney, *Memoirs* Vol. II, pp. 207, 209.

[20]Roberts, "Personnel and Practice, part 1, The Provinces, pp. 363, 369.

[21]Christopher Hill, "The Medical Profession and Its Radical Critics" in *Change and Continuity*, p. 165.

[22]Webster, *The Great Instauration*, p. 255.

[23]Pelling and Webster, *Medical Practitioners*, p. 235.

[24]Leonard Guthrie, "The Lady Sedley's Receipt Book, 1686, and other 17th Century Receipt Books,"*Proceedings of the Royal Society of Medicine*, 6 (1913): 150-170.

[25]Antonia Fraser, *The Weaker Vessel*, (London: Methuen, 1984) pp. 226-229. Fraser calls Anne Murray's efforts in 1650 "nursing", even though she describes her as having used "her own special balsam and plasters which she brought from England" and the fact that she treated large numbers of soldiers, some with advanced cases of gangrene, without any doctor or surgeon's help or supervision. J. Elise Gordon M.D. had also been guilty of the same type of distortion. See "Distinguised British nurses of the past," 2., "Lady Anne Halkett" *Midwife Health Visitor* (April 1975): 114-117.

[26]All of these examples from the seventeenth century are in Alice Clark, *Working Life*, pp. 263-265.

[27]Pelling, "Healing the Sick Poor," p. 128, 129. See also Pelling and Webster, "Medical Practitioners," pp. 222, 224 for women who were employed by sixteenth-century corporations for the treatment of illness.

[28]*Calendar of State Papers* 9 (1656) p. 219. Although some twentieth-century historians have called female practitioners "nurses", their seventeenth-century contemporaries did not make this mistake; the regulations also provided for nurses in a separate category. Scaldhead was an infection of the scalp with ringworm. (OED).

[29]J.S. Cockburn, (ed.) *Calendar of Assize Records, Sussex Indictments*. (London: Her Majesty's Stationery Office, 1975) p. 120. Sparmaceti was a fatty substance from sperm whale used in pharmacological preparations (OED).

[30]J. Cox, (ed.) *Dorset Folk Remedies* (Dorchester: Dorset Natural History and Archaeological Society, 1962) pp. 3, 4, 8.

[31]Philiatros, *Nature Exenterata:* (London, 1655; Thomason E1560), pp. 34, 37; Thomas, *Religion and the Decline of Magic*, p. 179; Verney and Verney, *Memoirs*, II, p. 279; W.M., *The Queen's Closet Opened* (London, 1655; Thomason E1519) p. 156 and "Index."

[32]Poynter and Bishop, (eds.) *Symcotts*. pp. 71-72, 55.

[33]Verney and Verney, *Memoirs*, II, p. 43. See also Cox, *Dorset Folk Remedies*; Paul Seaver, *Wallington's World* (Stanford: Stanford University Press, 1985) for the description of how a Mrs. Mason treated the six-month-old-child of Nehemiah Wallington who was having convulsions in 1626. She used "plasters", whose content is not known, applied to the infant's head, stomach and feet. (pp. 89, 90).

[34]Hoby, *Diary* pp. 101-127. Lady Hoby is generally acknowledged as the first female English diarist.

[35]Ibid., pp. 168, 100. There was also Lady Hoby's attempt at a surgical cure of the child born without an anus. See above, p. 9.

[36]Ibid., p. 255.

[37]Ibid., pp. 131, 168, 210.

[38]Ann Clifford, *Lady Ann Clifford, Countess of Pembroke, Domestic Diary 1616-*

1619, ed. V. Sackville-West (London: William Heineman Ltd., 1923): pp. xxiii, 26.

[39]Ibid., p. 12.

[40]Thornton, *Autobiography*, pp. 33-34.

[41]Ibid., p. 46.

[42]Ibid., p. 152.

[43]Ibid., p. 106.

[44]Searle, *Barrington Letters*, pp. 45, 202. It is interesting to note that one of the medical compendia which appeared several decades later speaks of "the old Lady of Oxfords oyl of Excester," possibly the same preparation used by Lady Barrington. See above, p. 47.

[45]Ibid., pp. 21, 202, 203.

[46]Ibid., p. 232. Ophthalmic diseases were apparently treated quite frequently by women practitioners, see below, p. 68. Also of interest is the fact that John Evelyn wrote of "supping with a gentlewoman called Everard that was a very great chymist'" See Gordon, "Women Practitioners," p. 566.

[47]Harley, *Letters*, p. 46. Brilliana sent bezoar stone or calculus found in the stomach or intestines of ruminants and aurum potabile or gold held in suspension in a volatile oil; both were believed to have medicinal properties. (OED).

[48]Ibid., p. 53.

[49]Ibid., p. 66. Mrs. Wilkinson and Hannah Woolley (see below) were headmasters' wives who assumed some responsibility for the treatment of their husbands' students, which suggests another avenue which could be explored in uncovering women practitioners.

[50]Ibid., p. 130. Angelica root was a root from an aromatic plant used in cookery and medicine. (OED).

[51]See Raach, *Directory*, pp. 111, 112. This shows 18 physicians in Oxford and a further 22 at the university for a total of 40 physicians.

[52]Quoted in Hanlon (Sister Joseph Damien), "These Be But Women," p. 379. Leonard Guthrie has noted that Lady Anne's prescriptions as well as those of her mother and grandmother were included in *The Queen's Closet Opened*. See Guthrie "The Lady Sedley's Receipt Book," p. 166. For some examples of Lady Anne's receipts see *The Queen's Closet Opened*, pp. 149, 168.

[53]Halkett, *Autobiography*, pp. 55, 56.

[54]Ibid., p. 33.

[55]Hutchinson, *Memoirs*, p. 265. The editors of Lucy's memoirs note that "the gentlewoman" may have been Lucy or her mother whom Lucy described as having "a great deal of skill which was very profitable to many all her life" (p. 21).

[56]Mary (Boyle) Rich, Countess of Warwick, *Autobiography*, pp. 153, 157.

[57]Guthrie, "Lady Sedley's Receipt Book," pp. 162, 166.

[58]A.W. Walker, *The Holy Life of Mrs. Elizabeth Walker*, (London, 1690; Wing W305), p. 177.

[59]Poynter and Bishop, *Symcotts*, pp. xx, xxi, 63, 70, 80, 81, 103.

[60]Gardiner, *Oxinden Letters*, p. 179.

[61]Jane (Meautys) Bacon, Lady Cornwallis, *Correspondence*, p. 179.

[62]Marmaduke Rawdon, *The Life of Marmaduke Rawdon of York, or Marmaduke Rawdon the Second of That Name*, ed. R. Davies (London: Camden Society Vol. 85, 1863) p. 85.

[63]Hanlon, "These Be But Women," pp. 379, 389.

[64]Josselin, *Diary*, p. 40.

[65]Ibid., p. 13.

[66]Ibid., p. 186; an issue was a cut or ulcer made to allow blood or other matter to escape (OED).

[67]Ibid., p. 346.

[68]Ibid., p. 221. This was in the tradition of physicians who thought they could diagnose illness through uroscopy, a practice which fell into disrepute as the century progressed. Josselin had already shown a considerable preoccupation with viewing his own urine (pp. 112, 116, 149).

[69]Ibid., pp. 191, 128, 473, 601. Pellitory was a plant whose pungently flavoured root was used as a local irritant or salivant as well as for treating toothache (OED).

[70]Guthrie, "Lady Sedley's Receipt Book," p. 164.

[71]Hannah Woolley, *Supplement to the Queen Like Closet* (London, 1680; Wing W3277).

[72]Ibid., all of the foregoing bibliographical information was taken from Wolley's lengthy "Forward." It was the qualification of "good judgement" that male critics often challenged. See below, p. 173.

[73]Ibid., pp. 15-24.

[74]Sarah Fell, *Account Book*, pp. 61, 75, 93, 383, 395, 493. Numerous references were made to Jannes Drink which was made of tumeric, saffron and ale.

[75]Ibid., pp. 142, 197.

[76]Ibid., pp. 249, 284.

[77]Ibid., pp. 113, 389, 493.

[78]Ibid., pp. 56, 274, 410. Another "ancient" remedy which the Fells used was mithridatum (pp. 189, 405). See also Cockram "Tribute to Sabine," p. 94.

[79]B. Blackstone, (ed.) *The Ferrar Papers* (London: Cambridge University Press, 1938) p. 32.

[80]See Thomas Cocke, *Kitchin-physick* (London, 1676; Wing C4792) who advocated "Diet" as the best "Physick and Physician" ("Dedicatory"). For an interesting comparison in the way sixteenth-century female artisans on the continent adapted their work to household constraints see Davis, "Women in the Crafts in Sixteenth-Century Lyon".

[81]As early as 1598, publications were disseminating the view that gentlewomen could be educated if they wished. See W.P., *The Necessarie, Fit and Convenient Education of a Young Gentlewomen* (London 1598, reprint New York: DaCapo Press, 1969); Samuel Torshell *Woman's Glorie, a Treatise Asserting the due Honour of that Sex and Directing wherein that Honour Consists* (London, 1645; Wing T1941). Both of the foregoing suggest that the most suitable reading material for women was the Holy Scriptures indicating that education for women should be directed more at her moral than intellectual betterment. For an extreme statement of the view that "virtue" was more desirable than education, see *The Mother's Legacy to her Unborn Child* (London, 1684; Wing J756). The author, Elizabeth Jocelin, was herself well educated. She urged her husband that if they had a daughter, she should be taught "good Housewifery, writing and good works" - although the emphasis was on humility, Jocelin did want her daughter to be literate. See also Robert H. Michel, "English Attitudes Towards Women 1640-1700" *Canadian Journal of History* 13 (1978): 36-60 for the view that gentlewomen were denied the classics, but they "learned English and perhaps French" (p. 50). David Cressy, *Literacy and the social order* has given a bleak picture of women's literacy noting that housewifery skills did not entertain the need for literacy. His viewpoint could be questioned in the face of evidence of the widespread use of receipt books, but again how many of these were

found in the hands of any but the upper class is uncertain. On the other hand, Cressy's book is relevant because he stresses the practicality of the growth of literacy. One did not need to be well-educated or literate to be a healer. See also above, p. 51, 52.

[82]Verney and Verney, *Memoirs*, I, pp. 8, 9; see also Christina Hole, *The English Housewife in the Seventeenth Century* (London: Chatto and Windus, 1953). Her chapter "Kitchen and Stillroom" makes the latter an integral part of every housewife's domain, "even more than the kitchen" (p. 70).

[83]Josselin, *Diary*, pp. 104, 191, 214.

[84]Hoby, *Diary*, pp. 134, 180. Women often referred to their special rooms where they carried out their distilling and preparation of medicines as "closets".

[85]Clifford in Hoby, p. 54.

[86]John Gerard, *The Herball or General Historie of Plants* (London, 1597).

[87]John Parkinson, *Paradis in Sole, paradisus terrestris* (London, 1629) and *Theatrum botanicum* (London, 1640); Poynter and Bishop, *Symcotts*, p. xx.

[88]Eleanor Sinclair Rohde, *The Old English Herbals* (London: Longmans, Green and Co., 1922).

[89]Poynter, "Nicholas Culpeper and his Books," pp. 161, 162.

[90]Josselin, *Diary*, pp. 218, 628.

[91]Hoby, *Diary*, p. 169.

[92]Fell, *Account Book*, p. 95.

[93]Fiennes, *Journeys*, pp. 27, 120, 226, 34.

[94]Ibid., p. 277. One of the two remedies for a cough which appear in Ann Blencowe's receipt book calls for "maidenhaire" as one of the ingredients (p. 50).

[95]Fiennes, p. 277.

[96]Cockram, "Tribute to Sabine", p. 68.

[97]Ibid., p. 69.

[98]Ibid., p. 70.

[99]Private communication from Dr. J.D. Alsop, citing Public Record Office, London, Prob 11/254, fos 150-1.

[100]Verney and Verney, *Memoirs* 2, p. 284. John Symcotts also mentioned a cure which a mother had successfully used to treat her child's umbilical hernia; she had taken it from "an old English physick book" (p. 80).

[101]Diana Astry, "Diana Astry's Recipe Book" ed. Bette Stitt *Publications of the Bedfordshire Historical Record Society* 37 (1957): 83-168. The terms recipe, receipt, and receit were used interchangeably throughout the period.

[102]Guthrie, "Lady Sedley's Receipt Book", pp. 161, 162.

[103]Patricia Crawford, "Attitudes to Menstruation in Seventeenth-Century England," *Past and Present* 91 (1981): 70.

[104]Doris Cook (ed., trans.), "An Elizabethan Guernseyman's Manuscript Book of Gardening and Medical Secrets," *Channel Island Annual Anthology* I (1972/3): 13-39.

[105]*Reports of the Royal Commission on Historical Manuscripts*, 3rd report, 121b. See also the 2nd report, 46b, for other medical receipt books.

[106]Thornton, *Autobiography*, p. 337. See also pp. 33-34.

[107]Verney and Verney, *Memoirs*, I, p. 227.

[108]Searle, *Barrington Letters*, p. 36.

[109]The three private receipt books were Diana Astry's (see above); Susanne Avery, ed. R.G. Alexander *A Plain Plantain. Country Wines, Dishes and Herbal Cures from*

a 17th Century Household M.S. Receipt Book (Ditchling, Sussex: S. Dominic's Press, 1922); Ann Blencowe, *The Receipt Book of Mrs. Ann Blencowe,* A.D. 1694. (London: Guy Chapman, 1925).

[110]The three compendia used were: Elizabeth Grey, Countess of Kent, *A Choice Manuall of Rare and Select Secrets in Physick and Chyrurgery* (London, 1653; Wing K311; Philiatros, *Nature Exenterata*; W.M., *The Queen's Closet Opened.*

[111]Graunt, *Bills of Mortality.* See the tables following page 80; these show a total of 44, 487 deaths from these ailments.

[112]This conclusion is supported by the present writer's detailed, unpublished study of Stuart midwifery.

[113]Astry, *Recipe Book,* p. 157.

[114]Ibid., pp. 143, 144.

[115]Avery, *A Plain Plantain,* p. 42; Astry, *Recipe Book,* p. 112. Astry possibly found the receipt in one of Culpeper's translations since she called it Culpeper's receipt for Dr. Stephen's water. Astry noted: "It is good for women in labour and brings away the after birth."; Guthrie, "Lady Sedley's Receipt Book," p. 152. Guthrie notes that the prescription for Dr. Stephen's water appeared in dispensatories as late as 1739.

[116]Thornton, *Autobiography,* p. 106.

[117]W.M., *Nature Exenterata,* p. 164.

[118]Ibid., p. 147.

[119]Kent, *A Choice Manuel,* p. 75. Hannah Woolley included the prescription in her *The Accomplish'd Lady's Delight,* p. 17. In the year of its publication (1653), Matthew Boone described the Countess of Kent's book as a pocket book which had all the things needful in it both for physic and surgery, approved by the best renowned doctors: private communication from Dr. J. D. Alsop, citing British Library, Sloane MS 1000, fo 62.

[120]Woolley, *The Accomplish'd Lady's Delight in Preserving, Physic, Beautifying and Cookery* (London, 1675; Wing 3268). The breadth of Woolley's accomplishments was demonstrated in her *Supplement to the Queen-Like Closet,* which contained home decoration hints, cookery recipes, instructions on how to starch lace and write letters for women wishing to engage in correspondence in a variety of settings, in addition to medical and surgical receipts.

[121]*Ibid.*

[122]Trye, *Mediatrix,* p. 104.

[123]Sarah Ginnor, *The Woman's Almanack* (London, 1659; Thomason E2140).

[124]Cook, "The Regulation of Medical Practice," p. 25.

[125]Even an innovative historian who rejects the approach and methods of the standard literature on the history of medicine has an unsupported and uncritical acceptance of the view that the seventeenth century witnessed a significant erosion of women's position in health care; see Hilda Smith, "Gynaecology and Ideology in Seventeen-Century England," *Liberating Women's History: Theoretical and Critical Essays* B.A. Carroll ed. (Urbana, Ill.: University of Illinois Press, 1976.)

[126]Cotta, *Ignorant and Unconsiderate Practisers of Physick,* p. 25. See also Michel, "English Attitudes Towards Women 1640-1700," pp. 47-49.

[127]Cotta, pp. 32, 33. The patient in this case survived. For an example of a conscientious, well-respected physician whose application of Galenical principles in treating a critically ill patient resulted in her death, see Poynter and Bishop *Symcotts,* p. 51.

[128]Ibid., p. 26.

[129]Ibid., p. 30. Cotta was particularly critical of measures such as imbibing cold liquids in hot weather.

[130] Ibid., p. 29, for a French physician's comments on women empirics see N. Z. Davis *Society and Culture in Early Modern France*, (Stanford U.P., 1975), p. 261.

[131]See above, p. 39, for Cotta's prime concern. In addition, see the records of the College of Physicians for prosecutions against women practitioners.

[132]See for example Anthony Wood, *The Life and Times of Anthony Wood*, ed. A. Clark, 5 vols. (Oxford: Historical Society, 1891-1907) 2, pp. 100-101, for the moving account of Wood's mother's death as the result of negligence on the part of her physician Dr. Edmund Dickenson. See also C. Goodall, *The Royal College of Physicians of London* (London, 1684; Wing G1091) for the case of Dr. Tenant, pp. 365-367; *The Diary of John Manningham* ed., John Bruce, (Camden Society, 1868. Reprinted New York: Johnson Reprint Corp., 1968). Manningham was a lawyer whose diary for the years 1602, 1603 tells of a surgeon who was arrested for killing "divers" women by "annointing them with quicksilver" (p. 23).

[133]John Sadler, *The Sicke Woman's Private Looking Glass* (London, 1636. Reprint Norwood, N.J.: Walter J. Johnson Inc., 1977), Frontispiece and opposite page. Sadler probably had good reason to feel threatened in view of the high number of women practitioners in Norwich. See Pelling, "Occupational Diversity".

[134]Tanner, *Hidden Treasures* "To the Reader" points 4 and 5.

[135]Christopher Bentley "The Rational Physician: Richard Whitlock's Medical Satires," *Journal of the History of Medicine and Allied Sciences* 29 (1974): 180-195.

[136]Ibid., pp. 190, 191.

[137]Banister, *A Treatise*, no pagination.

[138]Poynter and Bishop, *Symcotts*, p. 55.

[139]Ibid., pp. xx, 80, 81.

[140]Blockwich, *Anatomia Sambuci*, p. 164.

[141]An examination of medical literature directed to women leads to the conclusion that an important segment of society (authors, printers, physicians and surgeons) credited women, especially of the upper class, with a fair degree of literacy. See above, note 81 for a brief discussion of women's literacy.

[142]Leonard Sowerby, *The Ladies Dispensatory Containing the Natures, Vertues and Qualities of all Herbs and Simples usefull in Physick.* (London, 1651; Thomason E1258).

[143]Vicary, *The Surgions Directorie*, "Forward".

[144]A. Massaria, trans. R.T., *De Morbis Foemines. The Woman's Counsellor; or The Feminine Physitian* (London, 1657; Thomason G 416): 78.

[145]A.M., *A Rich Closet of Physical Secrets.* (London, 1652; Thomason E670 (1)). The title page noted that some of the "physical Experiments" had been presented to the late queen Elizabeth, again increasing its appeal to women of all classes.

[146]Philiatros, *Nature Exenterata*, Index.

[147]Robert Pemel, *Tractatus, De facultentibus Simplicium* (London, 1653; Thomason E721 (2)).

[148]Edward Poeton, *The Chyrurgions Closet* (London, 1630; Reprint New York: DaCapo Press, 1968).

[149]Thomas Collins, *Choice and Rare Experiements in Physick and Chirurgery* (London, 1658; Thomason E1887 (1)). Two years earlier, Robert Turner dedicated a tract which he had translated to Mrs. Elizabeth Creswell, a widowed gentlewoman who was evidently an accomplished medical practitioner at the popular level. See Moulton, trans. R. Turner, *The Compleat Bone-Setter* (London, 1656; Thomason

E1673 (1)).

[150]R. Bunworth, *The Doctresse: A plain and easie method of curing those diseases which are peculiar to women* (London, 1656; Thomason 1714 (21)); Kent, *A Collection... the Countess of Kent*; W.M. *The Queen's Closet*

[151]Thomson, *Galeno-Pale*. Earlier evidence of women's ownership of medical books can be found in a copy of Christopher Langton, *An Introduction into Physicke*, (1550), the inscription reads: "Jane Blackborn her Book, God Give her Grace on it to Looke." See also J. Vernon, *The Compleat Scholler* (London, 3rd ed., 1666; Wing V251). This book was inscribed "Penelope Dodington her Book. June the 3 1677." It is the biography of a physician's son who died at 12 years of age, and gives a great deal of insight into the role of religion and sickness. See above, chapter 3. The name "Joanna Henryson" is stamped on a book of medical prescriptions by Richard Beete (1691). Included in the book are prescriptions by Hans Sloane and Richard Mead in *Reports of the Royal Commission on Historical Manuscripts*, 5th report, p. 365 (a) no. 34.

[152]Biggs, *Mataeotechnia Medicinae*, p. 19.

[153]Starkey, *Nature's Explication*, pp. 141, 202 and 30. See also above, p. 47.

[154]Culpeper, *A Physical Directory*, "Introduction".

[155]N. Culpeper, *A Directory for Midwives: or A Guide for Women, In their Conception, Bearing and Suckling their Children*. (London, 1651; Thomason E1340 (1)). See also F.N.L. Poynter, "Nicholas Culpeper and his Books," p. 161.

[156]Culpeper in Hill, *Change and Continuity*, p. 164.

[157]Gervase Markham, *Country Contentments* (London, 1615. Reprint, Amsterdam: DaCapo Press, 1973), p. 54. At least nine more editions of "The English Housewife" which formed a part of this book appeared during the century. Ralph Josselin mentioned a cure from this book (p. 642).

[158]Richard Allestree, *The Ladies Calling*, (London, 1673; Wing A1141) "preface", pp. 56-57.

[159]Boyle, *The Works*, 2, p. 243.

[160]This information was obtained from the *Dictionary of National Biography*, sub. Thomas Hobbes. The original source is unfortunately not directly cited and has not been located. Note also Ashmole, *Autobiographical and Historical Notes*, p. 672.

[161]Verney and Verney, *Memoirs*, I, pp. 375-376. Dr. William Denton, Sir Ralph's brother-in-law and close personal friend is the physician in question.

[162]Ibid., II, pp. 207-209.

[163]Ibid., II, p. 279.

[164]Ibid., II, p. 43.

[165]Ibid., I, p. 362.

[166]Walter Yonge, *Diary*, p. xxiii. According to Yonge, during a trip to London, the rough roads between the D'Ewes' home in Devon and London upset the baby to such an extent that his strenuous crying resulted in the rupture. Perhaps curing ruptures in children was an area of female expertise, see above p. 73 for the names of two other women who treated the condition.

[167]Thornton, *Autobiography*, p. 164. A pearl in the eye was a kind of cataract according to the OED. Banister's treatise on diseases of the eye indicated that women commonly treated eye disorders. See also above p. 68.

[168]Ashmole, *Autobiographical and Historical Notes*, p. 453.

[169]Josselin, *Diary*, pp. 212, 278.

[170]A. Clark, *Working Life*, p. 257.

[171]Hutchison, *Memoirs*, p. 427.

[172]Fletcher, *A Country Community in Peace and War: Sussex 1600-1660.* (London: Longman, 1975), pp. 39, 42.

Notes to Conclusion

[1]See Webster, *The Great Instauration*, p. 316 as well as above, pp. 46, 48, 49. In addition, see Michael Hunter *Science and Society in Restoration England* Cambridge: Cambridge University Press, 1981) for the way in which the role of science in seventeenth-century England has been "overestimated" by historians (p. 193).

[2]E. Weil, "The echo of Harvey's De Motu Cordis (1628) 1628 to 1657," *Journal of the History of Medicine* 12 (1957): 167-74; G. Whitteridge, *William Harvey and the circulation of blood*, (London: Macdonald & Co. Ltd., 1971) pp. 149-173, 235.

[3]Christopher Hill, *The World Turned Upside Down* (Harmondsworth, Middlesex: Penguin, 1975) pp. 292, 297-300, 303-5, 362.

[4]There is some evidence of a shortage of surgeons to treat wounded soldiers and sailors, victims of the war, but the impact on popular medicine appears negligible. See *State Calendar—Commonwealth, 1640-1659*, passim.

[5]As a further evidence of continuity in medical practice, see Pelling and Webster's study of the sixteenth century, "Medical Practitioners" p. 235.

Selected Bibliography

Primary Sources

Allestree, Richard *The Ladies Calling*. Oxford, 1673; Wing A1141.

Ashmole, Elias. *Autobiographical and Historical Notes, Correspondence, etc.* Vol. 2 1617-1660. Oxford: Clarendon Press, 1966.

Astry, Diana. "Diana Astry's Recipe Book." Edited by Bette Stitt. *The Publications of the Bedfordshire Historical Record Society*. 37 (1957): 83-169.

Avery, Susanna. *A Plain Plantain, Country Wives' Dishes and Herbal Cures from a 17th Century Household M.S. Receipt Book*. Edited by R.G. Alexander. *Ditchling: S. Dominic's Press, 1922*.

B., M. *The Ladies Cabinet Enlarged and Opened*. London, 1654; Wing B135.

Bacon, Jane Cornwallis, Lady. *Private Correspondence of Jane Lady Cornwallis, 1613-44*. London: S. & J. Bentley, Wilson and Fley, 1842.

Bailey, Walter. *Two Treatises Concerning Eie-Sight*. Oxford, 1616; reprint ed., Norwood, N.J.: Walter J. Johnson Inc., 1975.

Banister, Richard.I *A Treatise of One hundred and Thirteene Diseases of the Eye*. London, 1622; reprint ed. New York: DaCapo Press, 1971.

Bartholinus, Thomas. *The Anatomical History of Thomas Bartholinus*. London, 1653; Thomason E1521 (2)

Baxter, Richard. *A Life of the Reverend Richard Baxter 1615-1691*. 2 vols. edited by Fredrick J. Powicke. London: Jonathan Cope Ltd., 1924-1927.

Bayfield, Robert. *Enchiridion Medicum: Containing the Causes, Signs and Cures of all those Diseases that do Chiefly affect the body of Man, divided into three Books*. London, 1665; Thomason E1563.

Bell, Susanna. *The Legacy of a Dying Mother*. London, 1673; Wing B1802.

Biggs, Noah. *Mataeotechnia medicinae Praxeos. The Vanity of the Craft of Physick*. London, 1651; Thomason E625 (17).

Blackstone, B. ed. *The Ferrar Papers*. London: Cambridge University Press, 1938.

Blencowe, Ann. *The Receipt Book of Mrs. Ann Blencowe, A.D. 1694*. London: Guy Chapman, 1925.

Blockwich, Martin. *Anatomia Sambuci: or the Anatomie of the Elder*. London, 1655; Thomason E1534 (2).

Bonham, T. *The Chyrurgions Closet*. Collected by Edward Poeton, London, 1630. Reprint ed. Amsterdam: Theatrum Orbis Terrarum Ltd., 1968.

Borde (or Boorde), Andrew. *Here followeth a compendyous regyment or a dyetary of helth*. London, 1542; S.T.C. 3379.

Boulton, S. *Medicina Magica Tamen Physica. Magical, but natural Physick or a Methodical Tractate of Diastatical Physick containing the general cures of all infirmities*. London, 1656; Thomason E1678 (2).

Boyle, Robert. *Robert Boyle, The Works.* edited by Thomas Birch. Hildesheim: George Olms Verlagsbuchhandlung, 1965.

Bradwell, Stephen. *Physick for the Sickness Called the Plague.* London, 1636. Reprint ed. Amsterdam: Theatrum Orbis Terrarum Ltd., 1977.

Brugis, Thomas. *Vade Mecum or a Companion for a Chyrurgion: fitted for times of peace or war.* London, 1641; Thomason E1357 (2).

Browne, Thomas. *Religio Medici.* London, 1643. Reprint ed. Menston, England: Scolar Press, 1970.

Bunworth, R. *The Doctresse: A plain and easie method of curing those diseases which are peculiar to women.* London, 1656; Thomason E1714 (2).

Burghall, Edward. *Diary of the Reverend Edward Burghall, Acton, Chester 1628-33.* Edited by T.V. Barlow. London: n.p., 1855.

A Catalogue of Valuable Books etc. London, 1689; Wing C1416.

Carew, Sir Richard. *Excellent Helps Really Found out, tried and had (where of the Parties hereafter mentioned are true and sufficient Witnesses), by a Warming Stone.* London, 1652; Thomason E802 (1).

Cartwright, Thomas. *The Diary of Dr. Thomas Cartwright, Bishop of Chester.* Edited by Joseph Hunter. Printed for the Camden Society, 1843. Reprinted., New York, N.Y.: Johnson Reprint Corporation, 1968.

Chamberlen, Peter. *A Voice in Rhama: or, The Crie of Women and Children.* London, 1646; Thomason E1181 (8).

––––– *The Porre Man's Advocate* London, 1649; Thomason E52 (1).

––––– *The Character of a Quack Doctor, or the Abusive practices of Impudent Illiterate Pretenders to Physick exposed.* London; 1676; Wing C1988.

Charleton, W. *Deliramenti Catarrhi or the Incongruities Impossibilities and Absurdities couched under the Vulgar opinion of Defluxions* London, 1650; Thomason E601 (6).

A Chymical Dictionary Explaining Hard Places and Words met with all in the Writings of Paracelsus, and other obscure authors. London, 1650; Thomason E604 (5).

Clifford, Lady Ann, Countess of Pembroke. *The Diary of Lady Anne Clifford.* Edited by Victoria Sackville-West. London: William Heinemann Ltd., 1923.

Clowes, William. *A Right Fruitfull and Approved Treatise for the Artificial Cure of Struma.* London, 1602: S.T.C. 5446. Reprint ed. Amsterdam: Theatrum Orbis Terrarum Ltd., 1970.

Cockburn, J.S., editor. *Western Circuit Assize orders 1629-1648.* London: Butler and Tanner Ltd. for the Royal Historical Society (London), 1976.

Coelson, Lancelot. *The Poor Man's Physician and Chyrurgion.* London, 1656; Thomason E1666 (2).

Cocke, Thomas. *Kitchen-physick or Advice to the Poor By Way of Dialogue* London, 1676; Wing C4792.

Collins, Thomas. *Choice and Rare Experiments in Physick and Chirurgery.* London, 1658; Thomason E1887 (1).

Cook, Doris, ed. "An Elizabethan Guernseyman's Manuscript Book of Gardening and Medical Secrets." *Channel Island Annual Anthology* 1 (1972-73): 13-39.

Cooke, James. *Supplementum Chirurgiae or the Supplement to the Marrow of Chyrurgerie.* London, 1655; Thomason E1516.

––––– *Mellificium Chirurgae or the Marrow of Chyrurgerie.* London, 1648; Wing C6012.

Cooke, John. *Unum Necessarium or The Poore Man's Case Being an Expedient to make Provision for all Poore people in the Kingdome.* London, 1647; Thomason E425 (1).

Cotta, John. *A Short Discoverie of the Unobserved Dangers of Severall sorts of ignorant and unconsiderate practicers of Physicke in England: Profitable not only for the deceived multitude and easie for their mean capacities, but raising reformed and more advanced thoughts in the best understanding with direction for the safest election of a physician in necessity.* London, 1612; S.T.C. 5833.

Cox, J. Stevens, ed. *Dorset Folk Remedies of the 17th and 18th Centuries.* Dorchester: The Dorset Natural History and Archeological Society, 1962.

Culpeper, Nicholas. *Culpeper's School of Physick.* London, 1659; Thomason E1739.

_____ *Culpeper's Last Legacy* London, 1655; Thomason E1464.

_____ *A New Method of Physick: or a short view of Paracelsus and Galen's Practice: in 3 Treatises.* London, 1654; Thomason E1475 (3).

_____ *The English Physitian Enlarged. With Three Hundred, sixty and nine medicines made of English herbs that were not in any Impression until this.* London, 1653; Thomason E1455 (1).

_____ *Galen's Art of Physick.* London, 1652; Thomason E1287 (3).

_____ *Semeiotica Uranica or an Astrological Judgement of Diseases.* London, 1651; Thomason E1360 (2).

_____ *A Directory for Midwives: or a Guide for Women. In their Conception, Bearing and Suckling Children.* London, 1651; Thomason E1340 (1).

_____ *A Physical Directory or a Translation of the London Dispensatory.* London, 1649; Thomason E576 (1).

Dickinson, Francisco. *A Precious Treasury of Twenty Rare Secrets, Most Necessary, Pleasant and Profitable for all Sorts of People.* London, 1649; Thomason E575 (25).

Dioscorides. *The Greek Herbal of Dioscorides.* Edited by Robert T. Gunther. Oxford: John Johnson at the University Press, 1933.

Du Bosc, Jacques. *The Compleat Woman.* Translated by N. N. London, 1639; S.T.C. 7266.

Duchesne, Joseph. *The Practise of Chymicall and Hermeticall physicke.* Translated by T. Timme. London, 1605; S.T.C. 7276.

Elkes, Richard. *Approved Medicines of Little Cost, to preserve health and also to cure those that are sick. Provided for the Souldiers Knap-sack and the Country mans Closet.* London, 1651; Thomason E1379 (2).

Englishe Traveller A Direction for the English Traviller. London, 1635. Reprint ed. New York, N.Y.: Da Capo Press, 1969.

Evelyn, John. *Diary of John Evelyn.* Edited by John Bowle. Oxford: Oxford University Press, 1983.

Fanshaw, Lady Ann. *Memoirs of Lady Ann Fanshaw.* London: John Lane the Bodley Head, 1907.

Fell, Sarah. *The Household Account Book of Sarah Fell of Swarthmoor Hall.* Edited by Norman Penney. Cambridge: Cambridge University Press, 1920.

Fiennes, Celia. *The Journeys of Celia Fiennes.* Edited by Christopher Morris. London: Cresset Press, 1949.

Fioravanti, Leonard. *Three Exact Pieces of Leonard Phioravanti, Knight, and Doctor in Physick* London, 1651; Thomason E1642.

Fontanus, Nicholas. *The Woman's Doctour; or, an exact and distinct Explanation of all such Diseases as are peculiar to that Sex with Choise and Experimentall Remedies against the same*. London, 1652; Thomason E1284 (2).

Forman, Simon. *Autobiography and Personal Diary*. Edited by J.O. Halliwell. London: Richards Printer, 1849.

Francesse, Peter. *Advertisement*. London, 1656; Thomason 669f20 (41)g.

The French Mountebank or an Operator Fit for these Present Times. London, 1643; Thomason E93 (20).

French, John. *The Yorkshire Spaw*. London, 1652; Wing F2175.

Galenus, C. *Galen's Method of Physick; or his Great Master Peece*. Translated by Peter English. Edinburgh, 1656; Thomason E1701.

Gardiner, Dorothy, ed. *The Oxinden Letters 1607-1642*. London: Constable and Company, 1933.

Gardiner, Edmund. *Phisicall and Approved Medicines, as well in meere Simples as Compound Observations*. London, 1611. Reprint ed. Amsterdam: Theatrum Orbis Terrarum Ltd., 1969.

Gayton, Edmund. *The Religion of a Physician*. London, 1663; Wing G416.

Gerard, John. *The Herball or General Historie of Plants* (1597). edited by Marcus Woodward as *Leaves from Gerards Herball*. London: Gerald Howe, 1931.

Gerbier, Charles. *Eloquium Heronium or the Praise of Worthy Women*. London, 1651; Wing G583.

Ginnor, Sarah. *The Woman's Alamanack*. London, 1659; Thomason E2140 (1).

Glisson, Francis; Bate, George; and Regemorter, A. *A Treatise of the Rickets Being a Disease Common to Children*. London, 1650; Thomason E1267.

Goodall, Charles. *The Colledge of Physicians Vindicated*. London, 1676; Wing G1090.

––––––– *The Royal College of Physicians of London. An account of their proceedings against empirics*. London, 1684; Wing G1081.

Graunt, John. *Natural and political observations made upon the bills of mortality*. London, 1662. Reprint ed. by Walter F. Willcox. Baltimore: John Hopkins Press, 1939.

Guidat, Thomas. *The Register of Bath*. London, 1694; Wing G2199.

Guillimeau, James. *Child-Birth, or, The Happy Deliverie of Women*. London, 1612. Reprint ed. Amsterdam: Theatrum Orbis Terrarum, 1972.

Halkett, Anne. *The Autobiography of Anne Lady Halkett*. Edited by J.G. Nichols. Printed for the Camden Society, 1875. Reprint ed. New York, N.Y.: Johnson Reprint Corporation, 1965.

Hall, John. *Select Observations on English Bodies: or Cures both Empiricall and Historicall, performed on very eminent persons in desperate Diseases*. Translated by James Cooke. London, 1657; Wing H356.

Harley, Brilliana. *The Letters of Brilliana Harley (1625-1643)*. Edited by T.T. Lewis. Printed for the Camden Society, 1854. Reprint ed. New York, N.Y.: Johnson Reprint Corporation, 1968.

Harvey, William. *Anatomical Exercitation, Concerning the Generation of Living Creatures. To which are added Particular Discourses of Births, and of Conceptions etc*. London, 1655; Thomason E1435.

––––––– *The Anatomcial Exercises of Dr. William Harvey Professor of Physick, and Physician to the Kings Majesty, Concerning the motion of the Heart and Blood*. London, 1653; Thomason E1477 (2).

Harward, Simon. *Phlebotomy: or, A Treatise of letting of Blood*. London, 1601. Reprint ed. Amsterdam: Theatrum Orbis Terrarum Ltd., 1973

Hawes, Richard. *The Poore-man's Plaster Box*. London, 1634; reprint ed. New York, N.Y.: Walter J. Johnson, 1974.

Heydon, Sir Christopher. *An Astrological Discourse with mathematical demonstrations, proving the powerful and harmonical influence of the planets and fixed stars upon elementary bodies, in justification of the validity of astrology*. London, 1650; Wing H1663.

Heywood, Oliver. *Life of John Angier of Denton*. Edited by E. Axon. Manchester: The Chetham Society, 1937; reprint ed. New York, N.Y.: Johnson Reprint Corporation, 1968.

Highmore, Nathaniel. *The History of Generation*. London, 1651; Thomason E1369.

Hinton, Sir John. *Memoirs of Sir John Hinton, Physitian in ordinary to His Majesties Person*. London: T. Bentley, 1814.

Hoby, Lady Margaret. *Diary of Lady Hoby*. Edited by Dorothy Meads. Boston and New York: Houghton Mifflin Company, 1930.

Hodges, Nathaniel. *Vindiciae Medicinae and Medicorum: or an Apology for the Profession and Professors of Physick*. London, 1665; Wing H2307.

Holland, P. *Regimen Sanitas Salerni or the Schoole of Salernes Regiment of Health*. Translated by P.H. London, 1649; Thomason E592.

Humble Petition of many thousands of Courtiers' Citizens', Gentlemen's and Tradesmen's wives etc. London, 1641; Thomason 669f4 (59).

Hunter, Richard, and MacAlpine, Ida, editors. "The Diary of John Causabon." *Proceedings of the Huguenot Society (London)* 21 (1966):31-57.

Hutchinson, Lucy. *Memoirs of the Life of Colonel Hutchinson*. 2 Vols. Edited by Julius Hutchinson. London: John C. Nimmo, 1885.

Irvine, C. *Medicina Magnetica: or the rare and wonderful Art of Curing by Sympathy*. London, 1656; Thomason E1578 (1).

Jocelin, Elizabeth. *The Mother's legacy to her Unborn Child*. London, 1684; Wing J756.

Jorden, Edward. *A Disease Called The Suffocation of the Mother*. London, 1603; reprint ed. New York: Da Capo Press, 1971.

Joseph, Harriet, ed. *Shakespeare's Son-in-Law: John Hall, Man and Physician*. Hamden, Conn.: Archon, 1964.

Josselin, Ralph. *Diary of Ralph Josselin 1616-1683*. Edited by Alan MacFarlane. London: Oxford University Press, New Series, 1976.

Kent, Elizabeth Grey, Countess of. *A Choice Manuall of Rare and Select Secrets in Physick and Chyrurgery fr. London, 1653; Wing K311*.

Lake, Rev. Edward. *Diary of the Rev. Edward Lake (1641-1704)* in Camden Miscellany Vol. I, 39. Printed for the Camden Society, 1847. Reprint ed. New York, N.Y.: Johnson Reprint Corporation.

Langton, Christopher. *An Introduction into Physicke, wyth an Universal Dyet*. London, 1550; S.T.C. 15204.

Levens, Peter. *The Path-Way to Health*. London, 1654; Thomason E1472.

Lloyde, Humfrey, translator. *The Treasuri of Helth*. London, 1550; S.T.C. 14652.

Lowe, Roger. *The Diary of Roger Lowe of Ashton-in-Makerfield, Lancashire, 1663-74*. edited by William R. Sachse. New Haven: Yale University Press, 1938.

Lupton, Thomas. *A Thousand Notable Things of Sundry Sorts, enlarged*. London, 1659; Thomason E1747.

M., A. *A Treatise Concerning the Plague and the Pox*. London, 1652; Thomason E670 (2).

M., W. *The Queen's Closet Opened*. London, 1655; Thomason E1519.

Makin, Bathsua. *An essay to revive the antient education of gentlewomen.* London, 1598. Reprint ed. Amsterdam: Theatrum Orbis Terrarum Ltd., 1969.

Manningham, John. *Diary of John Manningham, of the Middle Temple, and of Bradbourne, Kent, Barister at Law, 1602-1603.* Edited by John Bruce. Printed for the Camden Society, 1868. Reprint ed. New York, N.Y.: Johnson Reprint Corporation.

Markham, Gervase. *Country Contentments.* London, 1615. Reprint ed. New York: Da Capo Press, 1973.

Massaria, A. *De Morbeis Foemineis. The Womans Counsellour or The Feminine Physitian.* Translated by R.T. London, 1657; Thomason E1650.

(Menedemus, Dalepater.) *Lex Ex lex or the Downfall of the Law and the Gospell. Being a Warning-peece to the Colledge of Physitians or prodromous Discourse to a subsequent tract Entitled, Medice Curate ipsum.* London, 1652; Thomason E673 (20).

The Midwives Just Petition or a Complaint of dives good Gentlewomen of that Faculty. London, 1643; Thomason E86 (14).

Millwater, Lewis. *Cure of Ruptures in Man's Bodie. By Physical and Chirurgical Meanes and Medicines.* London, 1650; Thomason E625 (9).

Moffet, Thomas. *Healths Improvement: or, Rules Comprising and Discovering the Nature, Method and Manner of Preparing all sorts of Food used in this Nation.* London 1655; Thomason E835 (16).

Morellus, P. *The Expert Doctor's Dispensatory.* London, 1657; Thomason E1565.

Moulton, Friar. *The Compleat Bone-Setter, Wherein The Method of Curing broken Bones and Strains and Dislocated Joynts, together with Ruptures, vulgarly called Broken Bellyes, is fully demonstrated.* Translated by Robert Turner. London, 1656; Thomason E1673 (1).

Naworth, G. *A New Almanack.* London, 1644; Thomason E1181 (4).

The Necessarie, Fit and Convenient Education of a young Gentlewoman. London, 1598. Reprint ed. New York: Da Capo Press, 1969.

Nicholson, Marjorie Hope, ed.. *Conway Letters: the correspondence of Anne, Viscountess Conway, Henry More, and their friends, 1642-1648.* Oxford: Oxford University Press, 1930.

Nollius, Henry, *Hermetical Physick or the right way to preserve, and to restore Health.* Translated by Henry Vaughan. London, 1656; Thomason 1714 (2).

An ordinance for the relief and maintenance of sicke and maimed soldiers. London, 1643; Thomason E74913.

Overbury, Thomas. "Sir Thomas Overbury his Wife" in Alexander M. Witherspoon and Frank J. Warnke, eds. *Seventeenth Century Prose and Poetry*, 2nd ed. New York: Harcourt, Brace Jovanovich, 1982.

Paracelsus. *Of the Supreme Mysteries of Nature.* Translated by R. Turner. London, 1655; Thomason E 1567 (2).

Paré, Ambroise. *Three and Fifty Instruments of Chirurgery.* London, 1631. Reprint ed. Amsterdam: Theatrum Orbis Terrarum Ltd., 1969.

Pecquet, John. *New Anatomical experiments of John Pecquet of Deip.* London, 1653; Thomason E 1521 (2).

Pemell, Robert. *Tractatus de Simplicium Medicamentorum Facultatibus: A treatise of the nature and Qualities of Such Simples as are most frequently used in Medicines, Both Purging and Others.* London, 1652; Thomason E660 (8).

———. *De Morbis Capitis or Of the Chief internal Diseases of the Head.* London, 1649; Thomason E1300 (1).

Phaedro, George. *Physicall and Chemical Practise*. London. 1654; Thomason E1497 (2).

Philander, Eugenius. *Drinking of Bath Waters*. London, 1673; Wing P1984.

Philartis. *Culpeper Revived from the Grave To Discover the Cheats of the grand Imposter Call'd Aurum Potabile*. London, 1655; Thomason E487 (2).

Philiatros, F. *Nature Exenterata: or Nature Unbowelled By the most Exquisite Anatomizers of Her*. London, 1655; Thomason E1560.

Pierce, Robert. *Bath Memoirs*. Bristol: Printed for H. Hammond, Bookseller at Bath, 1697.

de Planis Campy, D. *A Treatise of Phlebotomy*. Translated by E.W. London, 1658; Thomason E1929 (1).

Pont, J. *A Generall Almanack*. London, 1646; Thomason E1171 (1).

Powell, Walter. *Diary of Walter Powell*. Edited by Joseph Bradney. Bristol: John Wright and Co., 1907.

Poynter, E.N.L. and Bishop, W.J. eds. *A Seventeenth Century Doctor and His Patients: John Symcotts, 1592-1662*. Streatley, Bedfordshire; the Bedfordshire Historical Record Society, 1951.

Primrose, James. *Popular Errours or the Errours of the People in Physick*. Translated by Robert Wittie. London, 1651; Thomason E1227.

Rawdon, Marmaduke. *The Life of Marmaduke Rawdon of York, or Marmaduke Rawdon the Second of the Name*. Edited by Robert Davies. Printed for the Camden Society 1863. Reprint ed. New York, N.Y.: Johnson Reprint Corporation, 1968.

Read, Alexander. *The Manuall of the Anatomy or Dissection of the Body of Man*. 4th ed. London, 1653; Thomason E1522 (1).

———— *Most Excellent and Approved Medicines and Remedies For Most Diseases and Maladies Incident to Man's Body*. London, 1651; Thomason E1301.

———— *A Treatise of the first Part of Chirurgerie etc. containing the methodical doctrine of Wounds: delivered in Lectures in the Barber-Chirurgeons Hall, upon Tuesdays etc*. London, 1638. Reprint ed. Norwood, New Jersey, Walter Johnson Inc., 1976.

A Rich Closet of Physical Secrets. London, 1652, Thomason 670 (1).

Rogers, John. *Some Account of Life and Opinions of John Rogers*. Edited by E. Rogers. London: Longmans Green, 1867.

Romney, Henry Sydney. *Henry Sydney, earl of Romney, 1641-1701*. Edited by R.W. Blencowe. London: H. Colburn,. 1843.

Rondeletius, William. *The Countrey-Man's Apothecary or a Rule by which Countrey-men may safely walke in taking Physicke not unuseful for cities*. London, 1649; Thomason E 1405.

Ross, Alexander. *Arcana Microcosmi or the Hid Secrets of Mans Body disclosed*. London, 1651; Thomason E1405.

Rosselin, E. *The Byrth of Man Kynde*. Translated by Thomas Raynold. London, 1540. S.T.C. No. 21154.

Rous, John. *Diary of John Rous* Edited by M.A. Everett Green. Printed for the Camden Society, 1856. Reprint ed. New York, N.Y.: Johnson Reprint Corporation, 1968.

Sadler, John. *Enchiridion Medicum or Enchiridium of the Art of Physick*. Translated by Robert Turner. London, 1657; Thomason E1678 (2).

———— *The Sick Woman Private Looking Glass*. London, 1636. Reprint ed. Amsterdam: Theatrum Orbis Terrarum Ltd., 1977.

Schroder, John. *ZOOVTIA or The History of Animals as they are useful in Physick and Chirurgery*. London, 1658; Thomason E1759 (1).

Searle, Arthur ed. *Barrington Family Letters 1628-1632*. London: Offices of the Royal Historical Society, University College, 1983.

Sennertus, D. *The Institutions or Fundamentals of the Whole Art both of Physick and Chirurgery*. Translated by N.D.B.P. London, 1656; Thomason E1568.

Sermon, William. *The Ladies Companion or the English Midwife*. London 1671; Wing S2628.

Simotta, G. *Planetary Houres and cures availabel to lay practitioners*. London, 1631. Reprint ed. Amsterdam: Theatrum Orbis Terrarum Ltd., 1971.

Smith, John. *A Compleat Practice of Physick Wherein is plainly described, the nature, Causes, differences, and Signs, of all Diseases in the Body of Man*. London, 1656; Thomason E1630.

Sowerby, Leonard. *The Ladies Dispensatory Containing the Natures, Vertues and Qualities of all herbs and Simples usefull in Physick*. London; 1651; Thomason E1258.

Stanhope, George. *Meditations and Prayers for Sick persons in the Christian's Pattern*. 2nd ed. London, 1700; Wing T947.

Starkey, George. *Nature's Explication and Helmont's Vindication or a short and sure way to a long and sound Life*. London, 1656; Thomason E1635 (2).

Stokes, Ethel ed. "Surrey Wills Proved in the Prerogative Court of Canterbury in 1611." *Surrey Archeological Collections* 35 (1924), pp. 39-48.

A Table of the Chymical, Medicinal and Chirurgical Addresses made to Samuel Hartlieb Esq. London, 1655; Thomason E1509 (2).

Tanner, John. *The Hidden Treasures of the Art of Physick: Fully Discovered in Four Books*. London, 1658; Thomason E1847.

Thompson, James. *Helmont Disguised or the Vulgar Errour of Impericalls and Unskilfull Practicers of Physick Confuted*. London, 1657; Wing T999.

Thomson, George. *Galeno-pale*. London, 1665; Wing T1023.

Thornton, Alice. *The Autobiography of Mrs. Alice Thornton of East Newton, Co. York (1627-1707)*. Edited by C. Jackson. Durham: Andrew and Company, 1875.

Thrasher, Will. *The Marrow of Chymical Physick or the Practice of Making Chymical Medicines*. London, 1679; Wing T1080.

Torshel, Samuel. *The Woman's Glorie, a Treatise Asserting the due Honour of the Sexe and Directing wherein that Honour Consists*. London, 1645; Wing T1941.

Trye, Mary. *Medicatrix or the Woman Physician*. London. 1675; Wing T3174.

Turner, R. *Paracelsus of the Supreme Mysteries of Nature*. London, 1655; Thomason E1567 (2).

Twysden, Isabella. "The Diary of Isabella, Wife of Sir Roger Twysden, Baronet of Royden Hall, East Peckham, 1645-1651." Edited by F.W. Bennett. *Archeologica Cantiana* 41(1939): 113-116.

Venner, Tobias. *Via recta ad vitam longam*. London, 1650; Thomason E605 (1).

————— *A Brief and Accurate Treatise, concerning the taking of the fume of Tobacco, which the very many, in these dayes, doe too licentiously use*. London, 1621. S.T.C. 24642.

Verney, Frances P. and Verney, M.M. *The Verney Memoirs*. 2 vols. London: Longmans, Green and Co., 1925.

Vernon, J. *The Compleat Scholler*. 3rd ed. London, 1666; Wing V251.

Vicary, Thomas. *The Surgions Directorie, For young Practitioners, In Anatomie, Wounds and Cures etc*. London, 1651; Thomason E1265.

_____ *The Englishmans Treasure.* 9th ed. published by William Bremer. London, 1641; Wing V334.

Vincent, T. *God's Terrible Voice in the City Two late dreadful judgements of Plague and Fire in London* London, 1667; Wing V440.

Walker, Anthony. *The Holy Life of Mrs. Elizabeth Walker.* London, 1690; Wing W305.

Walwyn, William. *A Touchstone for Physick, Directing by Evident Marks and Characters to such Medicines as without purgers, vomiters, bleedings, Issues, minerals; or any other disturbers of Nature.* London, 1667; Wing W693.

Ward, Rev. John. *Diary of the Rev. John Ward A.M.: Vicar of Stratford-Upon-Avon 1648-79.* Edited by C. Severn. London: Henry Colborn Pub., 1839.

Warwick, Mary Rich, Countess of. *Autobiography of Mary, Countess of Warwick. Edited by T. Crofton Croker. London: Richards, 1848, for the Percy Society.*

Wharton, George. *A New Almanack.* London, 1647; Thomason E1198 (2).

White, J. *A Rich Cabinet with Variety of Inventions.* London, 1651; Thomason E1295 72).

Williams, Ralph. *Physical Rarities Containing the Most Choice Receipts of Physick and Chyrurgerie. For the Cure of All Diseases incident to Man's Body.* London, 1651; Thomason E1302.

Williams, W. *Occult Physick.* London, 1660; Thomason E1737 (2)

Willis, Thomas. *A Plain and Easie Method for Preserving [By God's Blessing] those that are well from the Infection of the Plague, or any Contagious Distemper in the City, Camp, Fleet etc., and for curing such as are infected with it.* London, 1691; Wing W2852.

Winston, Thomas. *Anatomy Lectures at Gresham Colledge.* London, 1659; Thomason E1746.

Winter, Salvator. *A New Dispensatory of Fourty Physicall Receipts.* London, 1649; Thomason E573 (3).

_____ *Advertisement.* London, 1647; Thomason E826 (19).

Wood, Anthony A. *The Life and Times of Anthony Wood.* Edited by Andrew Clark. 5 vols. Oxford: Clarendon Press, 1891-1907.

Woodall, John, *The Surgions Mate.* London, 1617; S.T.C. 25962.

Woolley (Wolley), Hannah. *Supplement to the Queen Like Closet.* London, 1688; Wing 3287.

_____ *The Accomplish'd Lady's Delight in Preserving, Physick, Beautifying and Cookery.* London, 1675; Wing W3268.

Wright, Robert. *A Receipt to stay the plague; delivered in a sermon.* London, 1625; S.T.C. 26037.

Wynell, John. *Lues Venerea or a Perfect Cure of the French Pox: Wherein the Names, Nature, Subject, Causes and Signes of the Disease are handled* London, 1660; Thomason E1855 (2).

Yonge, Walter. *Diary of Walter Yonge Esq.* Edited by George Roberts. Printed for the Camden Society 1848. Reprint ed. New York, N.Y.: Johnson Reprint corporation, 1968.

Young, Sidney. *The Annals of the Barber Surgeons of London.* London: Blades East and Blades, 1890.

Government Documents

Great Britain. Public Record Office. *Calendar of Assize Records, James I, Sussex indictments.* Edited by J.S. Cockburn. London: Her Majesty's Stationery Office, 1975.

Great Britain. Public Record Office. *Calendar of State Papers, Domestic Series of the Reign of Charles I,* volumes 1-23 (1625-1649).

Great Britain. Public Record Office. *Calendar of State Papers, Domestic Series, Commonwealth.* Volumes 1-13 (1649-1659).

Great Britain. Historical Manuscripts Commission. *Reports of the Royal Commission on Historical Manuscripts.* Reports 3, 5, 6, 8 and 9.

Great Britain. Historical Manuscript Commission. *Rutland Mss.* volume 4.

Secondary Sources

Books and Theses

Ballard, George. *Memoirs of British Ladies, Who have been Celebrated for their Writing or Skill in the Learned Languages, Arts and Sciences,* 2nd ed. Oxford: n.p., 1752.

Berlant, Jeffrey L. *Profession and Monopoly: A Study of Medicine in the United States and Great Britain.* Berkeley: University of California Press, 1975.

Bier, A.L. *The Problem of the Poor in Tudor and Early Stuart England.* London: Methuen, 1983.

———. "The Social Problems of an Elizabethan Country Town: Warwick, 1580-90" in Peter Clark, ed. *Country Towns in Pre-Industrial England* New York: St. Martin's Press, 1981.

Bynum, W.F. and Porter, Roy, eds. *Medical Fringe and Medical Orthodoxy 1750-1850.* Beckenham, Kent: Croom Helm, 1987.

Cartwright, Frederick F. *A Social History of Medicine.* London: Longman, 1977.

Clark, Alice. *Working Life of Women in the Seventeenth Century.* London: Frank Cass and Co. Ltd., 1919. Reprint ed. Fairfield, N.J.: Augustus M. Kelley, 1978.

Clark, Sir George. *A History of the Royal College of Physicians of London.* 2 vols. Oxford: Clarendon Press, 1964.

Clark, Peter and Slack, Paul, eds. *Crisis and Order in English Towns 1500-1700.* Toronto: University of Toronto Press, 1972.

Coleman, D.C. *The Economy of England.* Oxford: Oxford University Press, 1977.

Cook, Harold John. "The Regulation of Medical Practice in London Under the Stuarts 1607-1704." Ph.D. Dissertation, University of Michigan, 1981.

Copeman, W.S.C. *Doctors and Disease in Tudor Times. London: William Dawson and Sons, 1960.*

Cressy, David. *Literacy and the Social Order.* Cambridge: Cambridge University Press, 1980.

Davis, Audrey B. *Circulation Physiology and Medical Chemistry in England 1650-1680.* Laurence, Kansas: Coronado Press, 1973.

Debus, Allen G., ed. *Medicine in Seventeenth Century England: a symposium held at U.C.L.A. in honour of C.D. O'Malley.* Berkeley: University of California Press, 1975.

———. *The English Paracelsians.* London: Oldbourne, 1965.

Donnison, Jean. *Midwives and Medical Men.* London: Heinemann, 1977.

Eccles, Audrey. *Obstetrics and Gynaecology in Tudor and Stuart England.* London: Croom Helm, 1982.

Ehrenreich, Barbara and English, Deirdre. *Witches, Midwives and Nurses: a history of women healers* 2nd ed. Old Westbury, New York: Feminist Press, 1973.

Fletcher, Anthony. *A Country Community in Peace and War: Sussex 1600-1660.* London: Longman, 1975.

Frank, Robert G. *Harvey and the Oxford Physiologists: Scientific Ideas and Social Interaction.* Berkeley: University of California Press, 1980.

―――― "The Physician as Virtuoso in 17th Century England" in B. Shapiro and R. Frank *English Virtuosi in the 16th and 17th centuries.* Berkeley: University of California Press, 1980, pp. 59-114.

Fraser, Antonia. *The Weaker Vessel Woman's Lot in Seventeenth-Century England.* London: Methuen, 1984.

Godfrey, Elizabeth [Jessie Bedford]. *Social Life under the Stuarts.* London: Grant Richards, 1904.

Grigg, David. *Population Growth and Agrarian Change: A Historical Perspective.* Cambridge: Cambridge University Press, 1980.

Haggard, H.W. *Devils, Drugs and Doctors: The Story of the Science of Healing from the Medicine Man to Doctor.* New York: Harper and Bros., 1929.

Hanlon, Sister Joseph Damien. "These Be But Women" in Charles H. Carter, ed. *From the Renaissance to the Counter Reformation.* New York: Random House, 1965.

Hole, Christina. *The English Housewife in the Seventeenth Century.* London: Chatto and Windus, 1953.

Hill, Christopher. *Change and Continuity in Seventeenth-Century England.* London: Weidenfeld and Nicolson, 1974.

―――― *The World Turned Upside Down.* London: Temple Smith, 1972; Penguin Books, 1975.

―――― *Intellectual Origins of the Revolution.* London: Clarendon Press, 1965.

―――― *Society and Puritanism in Pre-Revolutionary England.* London: Secker & Warburg, 1964.

―――― Lamont, W. and Reay, B. *The World of the Muggletonians.* London: Temple Smith, 1983.

Hughes, Muriel Joy. *Women Healers in Medieval Life and Literature.* Freeport, N.Y.: Books for Libraries Press, 1943.

Hull, Suzanne. *Chaste, Silent and Obedient: English Books for Women, 1475-1640.* San Marino, Ca.: Huntington Library, 1982.

Hunter, Michael. *Science and Society in Restoration England.* Cambridge: Cambridge University Press, 1981.

Illich, Ivan. *Limits to Medicine: medical nemesis, the expropriation of health.* Harmondsworth and New York: Penguin, 1977.

Jordan, W.K. *Philanthrophy in England 1480-1660.* London: George Allen and Unwin Ltd., 1959.

Kamm, Josephine. *Hope Deferred: Girl's Education in History.* London: Methuen and Co. Ltd., 1965.

Kanner, Barbara. *The Women of England: from Anglo-Saxon Times to the Present: interpretive bibliographical essays.* Hamden, Conn.: Archon Books, 1979.

Kealey, Edward J. *Medieval Medicus.* Baltimore, Md.: Johns Hopkins University Press, 1981.

King, Lester S. *The Road to Medical Enlightenment 1650-1695.* London: MacDonald, 1970.

Laslett, Peter. *The World We Have Lost.* London: Methuen and Company Ltd., 2nd ed. with corrections, 1979.

———— and Harrison, John. "Clayworth and Cogenhoe," in H.E. Bell and R. Lollard. *Historical Essays 1600-1750.* London: Adam and Charles Black, 1963.

MacDonald, Michael. *Mystical Bedlam: Madness, Anxiety and History in Seventeenth-Century England.* Cambridge: Cambridge University Press, 1981.

Mallett, Sir Charles Edward. *A History of the University of Oxford.* 3 vols. New York: Longmans Green and Co., 1924-1928.

Munk, William. *The Roll of the Royal College of Physicians of London: comprising biographical sketches.* 2nd ed. London: The College, 1878.

Newman, Sir George. *Interpreters of Nature.* Freeport, N.Y.: Books for Libraries Press, 1968.

Norsworthy, Laura. *The Lady of Bleeding Heart Yard. Lady Elizabeth Hatton 1578-1646.* London: John Murray, 1935.

Notestein, W. "The Englishwoman 1580-1650" in J.H. Plumb, ed. *Studies in Social History: a tribute to Trevelyan.* London: Longmans, Green, 1955.

Parry, Noel and Parry, Jose. *The Rise of the Medical Profession.* London: Croom Helm, 1976.

Patten, John. *English Towns 1500-1700.* Folkestone, Kent: Dawson: Archon Books, 1978.

Peachey, George C. *The Life of William Savory (surgeon) of Brightwalton.* London: J.J. Keliher & Co. Ltd., 1903.

Pollack, K. and Underwood, E.A. *The Healers: The Doctor then and now.* London: Nelson, 1968.

Pinchbeck, Ivy and Hewitt, Margaret. *Children in English Society,* 2 vols. London: Routledge and Kegan Paul, 1969.

Raach, John H. *A Directory of English Country Physicians 1603-1643.* London: Dawsons of Pall Mall, 1962.

Ramsey, Peter, ed. *The Price Revolution in Sixteenth-Century England.* London: Methuen and Co. Ltd., 1971.

Reiser, Stanley Joel. *Medicine and the Reign of Technology.* Cambridge: Cambridge University Press, 1978.

Richardson, R.C. *Puritanism in North-West England.* Manchester: Manchester University Press, 1972.

Robb-Smith, A.H.T. "Medical Education at Oxford and Cambridge Prior to 1850" in F.N.L. Poynter, ed. *The Evolution of Medical Education in Britain.* London: Pitman Medical Publishing Co. Ltd., 1966.

Rohde, Eleanor Sinclair. *The Old English Herbals.* London: Longmans, Green and Co., 1922.

Rowbotham, Sheila. *Hidden from History: rediscovering women in history from the 17th century to the present.* New York: Pantheon, 1974.

Rowland, Beryl. *Medieval Woman's Guide to Health: The First English Gynecological Handbook.* Kent, Ohio: Kent State University Press, 1981.

Seaver, Paul. *Wallington's World.* Stanford: Stanford University Press, 1985.

Silvette, Herbert. *The Doctor on Stage: Medicine and Medical Men in Seventeenth-century England.* ed. F. Butler. Knoxville: University of Tennessee Press, 1967.

Smith, Hilda. "Gynaecology and Ideology in Seventeenth-Century England," "Feminism and the Methodology of Women's History." both in Bernice A. Carroll, ed. *Liberating Women's History: Theoretical and Critical Essays.* Urbana, Ill.: University of Illinois Press, 1976.

Smith, Snell Donna. "Tudor and Stuart Midwifery." Ph.D. dissertation, University of Kentucky, 1980.

South, J.F. *Memorials of the Craft of Surgery in England.* ed. D'Arcy Power. London: Cassell and Company Limited, 1886.

Stone, Lawrence. *The Family, Sex and Marriage, in England 1500-1800.* Harmondsworth, Middlesex: Penguin Books, 1979.

Thomas, Keith. *Religion and the Decline of Magic.* London: Weidenfeld and Nicolson, 1971.

Underwood, E. Ashworth, ed. *Science, Medicine and History: Essays in Honour of Charles Singer.* 2 vols. London: Oxford University Press, 1953.

Upton, Eleanor Stuart. *Guide to Sources of English History from 1603-1660: In Early Reports of the Royal Commission on Historical Manuscripts.* 2nd ed. New York: Scarecrow Press, 1964.

Webster, Charles. *Health, Medicine and Mortality in the Sixteenth Century.* Cambridge: Cambridge University Press, 1979.

——— *the Great Instauration: Science, Medicine and Reform 1626-1660.* London: Duckworth, 1975.

Whitteridge, Gweneth. *William Harvey and the Circulation of Blood.* London: Macdonald & Co. Ltd., 1971.

Periodical Publications

Adamson, J.E. "The Extent of Literacy in England in the Fifteenth and Sixteenth Century." *The Library* N.S. 10 (1929): 163-193.

Allen, Phyllis. "Medical Education in 17th Century England." *Journal of the History of Medicine* 1 (1946): 115-143.

Allison, K.J. "An Elizabethan Village Census'." *Bulletin of the Institute of Historical research* 36 (May, 1963): 91-103.

Axtell, James. "Education and Status in Stuart England: the London Physician." *History of Education Quarterly* 10 (1970): 141-159.

Barlow, Frank. "The King's Evil." *English History Review* 95 (January, 1980): 3-27.

Barnet, Margaret C. "The Barber Surgeons of York." *Medical History* 12 (1968): 19-30.

Bates, Donald G. "Sydenham and the Medical Meaning of Method." *Bulletin of the History of Medicine* 51 (1972): 324-338.

Bentley, Christopher. "The Rational Physician: Richard Whitlock's Medical Satires." *Journal of the History of Medicine and Allied Sciences* 29 (1974): 180-195.

Best, Michael. "Medical Use of a Sixteenth-Century Herball: Gervase Markham and the Banckes Herball." *Bulletin of the History of Medicine.* 53 (1979): 449-458.

Bishop, P. James. "John Archer's 'Secrets Disclosed'." *Tubercle* (London) 38 (1957): 432-435.

Bishop, W.J. "Transport and the Doctor in Great Britain." *Bulletin of the Institute of the History of Medicine* 22 (1948): 427-439.

Bosanquet, Eustace F. "English Seventeenth-Century Almanacks." *The Library* 4th series, 10 (March, 1930): 361-397.

Brockbank, William. "Sovereign Remedies. A Critical Depreciation of the Seventeenth-century London Pharmacopoeia." *Medical History* 8 (1964): 1-14.

Brody, Steven A. "The Life and Times of Sir Fielding Gould: man midwife and master physician." *Bulletin of the History of Medicine* 52 (1978): 228-250.

Burns, Nesbitt. "A Woman Doctor of the 17th century." *British Medical Journal* 1 (1941): 124.

Butler, William. "A Physician between two ages." *Medical History* 21 (1977): 434-445; 22 (1978): 417-430.

Charlton, Christopher. "A Midwife's Certificate." *Local Population Studies* 4 (1970): 56-58.

Cockram, E. Joyce. "Tribute to Sabine." *Journal of the Medical Women's Federation* 43 (1961): 86-96.

Coley, Noel G. "Cures without Care; Chymical physicians and mineral waters in Seventeenth-Century English Medicine." *Medical History* 23 (1979): 191-214.

Colwell, Hector A. "Lionel Lockyer" *Proceedings of the Royal Society of Medicine* 8 (1914): 126-134.

Cranfield, Paul A. "A Seventeenth Century View of Mental Deficiency and Schizophrenia: Thomas Willis on 'Stupidity or Foolishness'." *Bulletin of the History of Medicine* 35 (1961): 291-316.

Crawford, Patricia. "Attitudes to Menstruation in Seventeenth-Century England." *Past and Present* 91 (May, 1981): 47-73.

Crellin, J.K. and Scott, J.R. "Lionel Lockyer and his pills." *International Congress of the History of Medicine* 2 (Sept. 1972): 1182-1186.

Davis, Natalie Zemon. "Women in the Crafts in Sixteenth-Century Lyon." *Feminist Studies* 8 (1982): 46-80.

Debus, Allen G. "Some Comments on the Contemporary Helmontian Renaissance." *Ambix* 19 (1972):145-150.

Dewhurst, Kenneth. "Thomas Sydenham (1624-1689) Reformer of Clinical Medicine." *Medical History* 6 (1962): 101-118.

———— "Some Letters of Charles Goodall (1642-1712) to Locke, Sloane and Sir Thomas Millington." *Journal of the History of Medicine* 17 (1962): 487-508.

Dick, Hugh. "Students of Physical and Astrological Medicine in the Age of Science." *Journal of the History of Medicine and Allied Sciences* 1 (1946) No. 1, pp. 300-315; no. 3, pp. 419-433.

Forbes, Thomas. "The Registration of English Midwives in the sixteenth and seventeenth centuries." *Medical History* 8 (1964): 235-244.

Frank, Robert G. "The John Ward Diaries: Mirror of Seventeenth-century Science and Medicine." *Journal of the History of Medicine* 29 (1974): 147-179.

Frost, Kate. "John Donne's Devotions, an Early Record of Epidemic Typhus." *Journal of the History of Medicine and Allied Sciences* 31 (1976): 421-430.

———— "Prescription and Devotion: The Reverend Doctor Donne and the Learned Doctor Mayerne: two Seventeenth-century records of epidemic typhus." *Medical History* 22 (1978): 408-416.

Goldstein, Leba M. "The Life and Death of John Lambe." *Guildhall Studies in London History* 6 (Oct. 1979): 19-32.

Gordon, J. Elise. "Some Women Practitioners of Past Centuries." *Practitioner* 208 (1972): 561-67.

———— "Distinguished British Nurses of the Past." *Midwife Health Visitor* 2 (March, 1975): 77-8, (May, 1975): 139-142.

Guthrie, Leonard. "The Lady Sedley's Receipt Book, 1686 and other Seventeenth-century Receipt Books." *Proceedings of the Royal Society of Medicine* 6 (1913): 150-170.

Guy, John R. "The Episcopal Licensing of Physicians, Surgeons and Midwives." *Bulletin of the History of Medicine* 56 (1982): 528-542.

126   Popular Medicine in Seventeenth-Century England

Halliday, F.E. "Sir Richard Carewe's 'Book'." *Practitioner* 176 (1956): 543-9.

Harris, George. "Domestic Everyday Life Manners and Customs of this Country, from the Earliest Period to the End of the Eighteenth Century." *Transactions of the Royal Historical Society* 9 (1881): 224-53.

Harrower, Kate. "Mouse pie" [Letter on the use of mouse to cure enuresis and diabetes]. *British Medical Journal* 2 (1962): 994.

Hill, Brian. "Medical Imposters." *History of Medicine* 2 (1970): 7-11.

Hill, Christopher. "The Religion of Gerrard Winstanley." *Past and Present Supplement* 5 (1979).

Imlof, A.E. "Social and Medical History; methodological problems in Interdisciplinary quantitative research." *Journal of Interdisciplinary History* (Winter 1977): 493-8.

Jacob, Margaret. "Science and Social Passion: The Case of Seventeenth-Century England." *Journal of the History of Ideas* 43 (1982): 331-9.

Jacobs, J.P. "Robert Boyle and Subversive Religion in the Early Restoration" *Albion* 6 (1974): 275-93.

Jones, Gordon W. "A Relic of the Golden Age of Quackery: What Read Wrote." *Bulletin of the History of Medicine* 37 (1963): 226-238.

Kargon, Robert. "John Graunt, Francis Bacon and the Royal Society: The Reception of Statistics." *Journal of the History of Medicine.* 18 (1963): 337-348.

Keevil, J.J. "The Seventeenth-Century English Medical Background." *Bulletin of the History of Medicine* 31 (1957): 408-424.

Kerling, Nellie. "A Seventeenth Century Hospital Matron: Margaret Blague." *London and Middlesex Archeological Society Transactions* 22 (1970): 30-36.

Kocher, P.H. "The Idea of God in Elizabethan Medicine." *Journal of the History of Ideas* 11 (1950): 3-29.

Krivastsy, Peter. "William Westmacott's 'Memorablia': the education of a Puritan country physician." *Bulletin of the History of Medicine* 49 (1975): 331-8.

Larkey, S.V. "Public Health in Tudor England." *American Journal of Public Health* 24 (1935): 1099-1102.

Le Fanu, W.R. "A North Riding Doctor in 1609." *History of Medicine* 5 (1961): 178-188.

Levy, Hermann. "The Economic History of Sickness and Medical Benefit before the Puritan Revolution." *Economic History Review* 13 (1943): 42-57.

Matossian, Mary Kilborne. "Mold poisoning: an unrecognized English Health Problem, 1550-1800." *Medical History* 25 (1981): 73-84.

Matthews, Leslie G. "Licensed Mountebanks in Britain." *Journal of the History of Medicine* 19 (1964): 30-45.

Menzies, Walter. "Alexander Read, Physician and Surgeon, 1580-1641: his Life, Works and Library." *The Library* 4th ser. 12 (1932): 46-74.

Merton, Robert K. "Science, Technology and Society in Seventeenth Century England." *Osiris* 4 (1938): 360-362.

Michel, Robert H. "English Attitudes Towards Women 1640-1700." *Canadian Journal of History* 13 (April, 1978): 36-60.

McLaren, D. "Nature's Contraceptive: Wet Nursing and Prolonged Lactation: the case of Chesham, Buckinghamshire, 1578-1601." *Medical History* 23 (1979): 426-441.

Nutton, Vivian. "Dr. Butler Revisited." *Medical History* 22 (1978): 417-30.

Ober, William B. "Noble Quacksalver: The Earl of Rochester's Merry Prank." *History of Medicine* 5 (1973): 24-26.

O'Malley, C.D. "John Evelyn and Medicine." *Medical History* 12 (1968): 219-31.

Owen, Gilbert. "The Famous Case of Lady Anne Conway." *Annals of Medical History* 9 (1937): 567-71.

Pagel, Walter. "Van Helmont's Concept of Disease: To be or not to be? The Influence of Paracelsus." *Bulletin of the History of Medicine.* 46 (1972): 419-454.

Pelling, Margaret. "Healing the Sick Poor: Social Policy and Disability in Norwich 1550-1640." *Medical History* 29 (1985): 115-137.

_____ "Occupational Diversity: Barber Surgeons and the Trades of Norwich 1550-1640." *Bulletin of the History of Medicine* 56 (1982): 484-511.

_____ "A Survey of East Anglian Medical practitioners 1500-1640." *Local Population Studies* 25 (1980): 54-5.

Phelps-Brown, E.H. and Hopkins, Sheila V. "Seven Centuries of Building Wages." *Economica* 22 (1955): 195-206.

Plomer, H.R. "English Almanacs and Almanac-makers of the Seventeenth Century." *Notes and Queries.* 6th series 12 (1885) pp. 243, 244, 323, 324, 383, 384, 462-463.

Porter, Roy. "Was There a Medical Enlightenment in Eighteenth Century England?" *British Journal for Eighteenth-Century Studies* 5 (1982): 49-63.

_____ "Quacks and Doctors: One Man's herb, another man's medicine." *The Listener* (June 23, 1983) 14-16.

_____ "The Rage of Party: A Glorious Revolution in English Psychiatry." *Medical History* 27 (1983): 35-50.

_____ "Lay Medical Knowledge in the Eighteenth Century: The Evidence of the 'Gentleman's Magazine'." *Medical History* 29 (1985): 133-168.

Power, Sir D'Arcy. "The Birth of Mankind or the Woman's Book: A Bibliographical Study." *The Library* 4th series, 8 (1927): 1-37.

_____ "Fees of our Ancestors" *Lancet* 1 (Feb 7, 1920): 339-40.

Poynter, F.N.L. "Nicholas Culpeper and his Books." *Journal of the History of Medicine* 17 (1962): 155-67.

Raach, John H. "Five Early Seventeenth-Century English Country Physicians." *Journal of the History of Medicine* 20 (1965): 213-225.

Ramsey, Matthew. "Medical Power and Popular Medicine: Illegal Healers in Nineteenth-Century France." *Journal of Social History* 10 (1976): 560-87.

Richardson, R.G. "Dr. John Hall, Shakespeare's Son-in-law." *Practitioner* (April, 1981): 593-95.

Roberts, R.S. "The Personnel and Practice of Medicine in Tudor and Stuart England" *Medical History* 6 (1962): 363-382 and 8 (1964): 217-34.

_____ "Jonathan Goddard." *Medical History* 8 (1964): 190-91.

Sanguine, Eric. "The Private Libraries of Tudor Doctors." *Journal of the History of Medicine* 33 (1978): 167-84.

Schoneveld. C.W. "Sir Thomas Browne and Leiden University 1633." *English Language Notes* 19 (1982): 335-59.

Schnucker, R.V. "The English Puritans and Pregnancy, Delivery and Breast Feeding." *History of Childhood Quarterly* (Spring, 1974): 637-58.

Shaw, Batty A. "Sir Thomas Browne." *British Medical Journal* 285 (1982): 40-2.

Silvette, Herbert. "On Quacks and Quackery in Seventeenth-century England." *Annals of Medical History* 3rd ser. 1 (1939): 239-251.

Simmons, Judith. "Publications of 1623." *The Library* 5th ser. 21 (1966): 207-222.

Siraisi, Nancy G. "Some Current Trends in the Study of Medicine." *Renaissance Quarterly* 37 (Winter, 1984): 585-600.

Stannard, Jerry. "Materia Medica in the Locke-Clarke Correspondence." *Bulletin of the History of Medicine* 37 (1963): 201-5.

Sisson, C.J. "Shakespeare's Helena and Dr. William Harvey." *Essays and Studies* (1960): 1-20.

Thirsk, Joan. "Younger Sons in the Seventeenth Century." *History* 44 (1969): 358-377.

Tourney, Garfield. "The Physician and Witchcraft in Restoration England." *Medical History* 16 (1972): 143-55.

Urbang, G. "The Mystery about the First English (London) Pharmacopoeia (1618)." *Bulletin of the Institute of the History of Medicine* 12 (1942): 304-13.

Weigall, Rachel. "An Elizabethan Woman: The Journal of Lady Mildmay." *Quarterly Review* 215 (1911): 119-38.

Weil, E. "The Echo of Harvey's De Motu Cordis (1628) 1628 to 1657." *Journal of the History of Medicine* 12 (1957): 167-174.

Whittet, T.D. "The Apothecary in Provincial Gilds." *Medical History* 8 (1964): 245-73.

Wilmott Dobbie, B.M. "An Attempt to Estimate the True Rate of Maternal Mortality, Sixteenth to Eighteenth Centuries." *Medical History* 26 (1982): 79-90.

Worden, Blair. "Providence and Politics in Cromwellian England." *Past and Present* 109 (Nov. 1985): 56-99.

Index

This book is useful for historical
reasons only. It does not contain
current medical information.